Pounds and Inches Pocket Reference

Simeons' Manuscript with Charts,
Checklists, and Resources for the HCG Diet

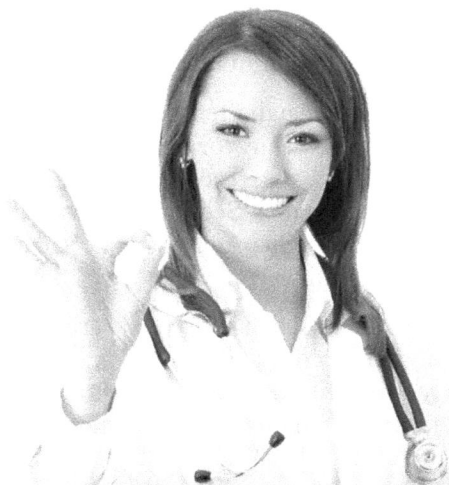

Harmony
Clearwater Grace

Pounds and Inches Pocket Reference

Dear hCG Diet Friends,

I've gotten lots of feedback from my readers over the years that the HCG Diet Made Simple book has been in print form. One of the most common comments that I hear is that the book is too large to carry in a pocket of purse, in order to be able to quickly refer to it when shopping or away from home.

Another comment is that people would like to carry Dr. Simeons' original manuscript text for easy reference as well, so it is included in this edition of the Pocket Reference.

One of the most important things to me is that my information be able to be used effectively to make an HCG Dieter's experience of weight release the best that it can possibly be. For that reason, I am publishing this new smaller abridged Pocket Reference to provide that portable data that so many have requested.

Blessings with Love,

Harmony

P.S. Please email me when you have reduced below 200 pounds, if you start out above that, so that I can personally tell you, "Welcome to ONE-derland! Onward and downward!! (on the scale, that is)." Any other major milestone emails are also happily welcomed!

P.P.S. Always remember: You DESERVE to be thin and healthy!

About the Author

Harmony Clearwater Grace, author of the bestselling book _HCG Diet Made Simple_, continues her work by helping those who need to carry an HCG Diet pocket reference to be successful, with her newest book, Pound and Inches Pocket Reference: Simeons' Manuscript with Charts, Checklists, and Resources for the HCG Diet.

Harmony is also the author of _The HCG Diet Book of Secrets_, your guide to staying slim forever after the HCG Diet.

Harmony is a moderator of an HCG Dieters support group with over 30,000 members. Over the last few years, she has seen, researched, and answered the questions that all HCG Dieters ask about how to do the Simeons HCG protocol optimally. She herself has lost 55 pounds with HCG dieting and wishes to share what she has learned about it with you. This controversial diet is the only one to allow her to lose weight in almost ten years of obesity, after the majority of her life was spent naturally underweight. After finding this HCG miracle, she is devoted to helping all of the overweight and obese to a normal healthy weight, either for the first time, or once again. Her vision is to be a catalyst to a complete turnaround of the current obesity epidemic through her work.

Wholesale Pricing

If you operate a clinic with an HCG Diet program, an HCG Diet blog, health website, or bookstore, become an affiliate and earn commissions on referred sales of this book. To post a link on your website or inquire about wholesale pricing or distribution of the print book, contact us at

affiliates@hcgdietmadesimple.com or

wholesalepurchases@hcgdietmadesimple.com.

PLEASE NOTE: The law requires this statement be posted:

The FDA has not approved hCG for weight loss and there is no substantial evidence that hCG is effective in the treatment of obesity.

I do, of course, respectfully disagree with the FDA.

Table of Contents

Acknowledgements

Whenever possible, I cite references to support my opinions, sometimes from the Pounds and Inches manuscript itself and sometimes from the internet or clinical studies. When I cite references from the internet, I include a shortened URL using TinyURLs throughout this book for your convenience in using the URL links with minimum keystrokes. These URL references are not necessary for full understanding of my reasoning, but provide the actual research links that I used, in case you would like to read further background. As time goes on, the websites for those URLs may be changed or deleted altogether, as the internet is not a static reference, nor under my direct control in terms of how it changes. If you find that any URL link in this book no longer works, I apologize in advance, for these conditions beyond my control. If reported to me as a broken link, I will update the TinyURLs according to page number at this Web page:

http://www.hcgdietmadesimple.com/Updates.

If you have any questions or concerns about the data in this book, I am always available through email to offer whatever help and support that I can. I am also very interested in hearing your story and how this information has helped you. Please be aware, however, that I am not a medical professional and that I cannot answer medical questions.

Please email your comments, questions that are not answered in this book, and stories of your successful weight reduction to:

hcgdietmadesimple@gmail.com.

We only recommend products that we've either personally checked out ourselves or that come from people we know and trust. For doing so, we may receive compensation. Results are unique. Your results may vary.

.

Abbreviations Used in This Book

Dr. S = A.T.W. Simeons, M.D.

VLCD = Very Low Calorie Diet

LIW = Last Injection Weight

LSDW = Last Sublingual Dose Weight

P1 = Phase 1 = Detox/cleanses before the diet

P2 = Phase 2 = hCG plus 500-calorie diet, followed by 72 hours of 500 calories after last dose of hCG

P3 = Phase 3 = Three weeks of no sugar and no starch

P4 = Phase 4 = Three additional weeks after the first round (increased periods of time after subsequent rounds) of gradually re-introducing sugar/starch into the diet in small amounts, always controlled by morning weighing

Scan this code with your Smartphone to join my smaller private support group.

Click the blue "Join this Group" at the top right of the webpage. Or you can visit: http://goo.gl/idjQf

POUNDS AND INCHES

A New Approach to Obesity

BY

A.T.W. SIMEONS M.D.

SALVATOR MUNDI INTERNATIONAL HOSPITAL

00152 - ROME

VIALE MURA GIANICOLENSI, 77

FOREWORD

This book discusses a new interpretation of the nature of obesity, and while it does not advocate yet another fancy slimming diet it does describe a method of treatment which has grown out of theoretical considerations based on clinical observation.

What I have to say is an essence of views distilled out of forty years of grappling with the fundamental problems of obesity, its causes, its symptoms, and its very nature. In these many years of specialized work thousands of cases have passed through my hands and were carefully studied. Every new theory, every new method, every promising lead was considered, experimentally screened and critically evaluated as soon as it became known. But invariably the results were disappointing and lacking in uniformity.

I felt that we were merely nibbling at the fringe of a great problem, as, indeed, do most serious students of overweight. We have grown pretty sure that the tendency to accumulate abnormal fat is a very definite metabolic disorder, much as is, for instance, diabetes. Yet the localization and the nature of this disorder remained a mystery. Every new approach seemed to lead into a blind alley, and though patients were told that they are fat because they eat too much, we believed that this is neither the whole truth nor the last word in the matter.

Refusing to be side-tracked by an all too facile interpretation of obesity, I have always held that overeating is the result of the disorder, not its cause, and that we can make little headway until we can build for ourselves some sort of theoretical structure with which to explain the condition. Whether such a structure represents the truth is not important at this moment. What it must do is to give us an intellectually satisfying interpretation of what is happening in the obese body. It must also be able to withstand the onslaught of all hitherto known clinical facts and furnish a hard background against which the results of treatment can be accurately assessed.

To me this requirement seems basic, and it has always been the center of my interest. In dealing with obese patients it became a habit to register and order every clinical experience as if it were an odd looking piece of a jig-saw puzzle. And then, as in a jig saw puzzle, little clusters of fragments began to form, though they seemed to fit in nowhere. As the years passed these clusters grew bigger and started to amalgamate until, about sixteen years ago, a complete picture became dimly discernible. This picture was, and still is, dotted with gaps for which I cannot find the pieces, but I do now feel that a theoretical structure is visible as a whole.

With mounting experience, more and more facts seemed to fit snugly into the new framework, and when then a treatment based on such speculations showed consistently satisfactory results, I was sure that some practical advance had been made, regardless of whether the theoretical interpretation of these results is correct or not.

The clinical results of the new treatment have been published in scientific journal[1] and these reports have been generally well received by the profession, but the very nature of a scientific article does not permit the full presentation of new theoretical concepts nor is there room to discuss the finer points of technique and the reasons for observing them.

During the 16 years that have elapsed since I first published my findings, I have had many hundreds of inquiries from research institutes, doctors and patients. Hitherto I could only refer those interested to my scientific papers, though I realized that these did not contain sufficient information to enable doctors to conduct the new treatment satisfactorily. Those who tried were obliged to gain their own experience through the many trials and errors which I have long since overcome.

Doctors from all over the world have come to Italy to study the method, first hand in my clinic in the Salvator Mundi International Hospital in Rome. For some of them the time they could spare has been too short to get a full grasp of the technique, and in any case the number of those whom I have been able to meet personally is small compared with the many requests for further detailed information which keep coming in. I have tried to keep up with these demands by correspondence, but the volume of this work has become unmanageable and that is one excuse for writing this book.

In dealing with a disorder in which the patient must take an active part in the treatment, it is, I believe, essential that he or she have an understanding of what is being done and why. Only then can there be intelligent cooperation between physician and patient. In order to avoid writing two books, one for the physician and another for the patient – a prospect which would probably have resulted in no

---

[1] A list of references to the more important articles is given at the end of this booklet.

book at all – I have tried to meet the requirements of both in a single book. This is a rather difficult enterprise in which I may not have succeeded. The expert will grumble about long-windedness while the lay-reader may occasionally have to look up an unfamiliar word in the glossary provided for him.

To make the text more readable I shall be unashamedly authoritative and avoid all the hedging and tentativeness with which it is customary to express new scientific concepts grown out of clinical experience and not as yet confirmed by clear-cut laboratory experiments. Thus, when I make what reads like a factual statement, the professional reader may have to translate into: clinical experience seems to suggest that such and such an observation might be tentatively explained by such and such a working hypothesis, requiring a vast amount of further research before the hypothesis can be considered a valid theory. If we can from the outset establish this as a mutually accepted convention, I hope to avoid being accused of speculative exuberance.

THE NATURE OF OBESITY

Obesity a Disorder

As a basis for our discussion we postulate that obesity in all its many forms is due to an abnormal functioning of some part of the body and that every ounce of abnormally accumulated fat is always the result of the same disorder of certain regulatory mechanisms. Persons suffering from this particular disorder will get fat regardless of whether they eat excessively, normally or less than normal. A person who is free of the disorder will never get fat, even if he frequently overeats.

Those in whom the disorder is severe will accumulate fat very rapidly, those in whom it is moderate will gradually increase in weight and those in whom it is mild may be able to keep their excess weight stationary for long periods. In all these cases a loss of weight brought about by dieting, treatments with thyroid, appetite-reducing drugs, laxatives, violent exercise, massage, baths, etc., is only temporary and will be rapidly regained as soon as the reducing regimen is relaxed. The reason is simply that none of these measures corrects the basic disorder.

While there are great variations in the severity of obesity, we shall consider all the different forms in both sexes and at all ages as

16

always being due to the same disorder. Variations in form would then be partly a matter of degree, partly an inherited bodily constitution and partly the result of a secondary involvement of endocrine glands such as the pituitary, the thyroid, the adrenals or the sex glands. On the other hand, we postulate that no deficiency of any of these glands can ever directly produce the common disorder known as obesity.

If this reasoning is correct, it follows that a treatment aimed at curing the disorder must be equally effective in both sexes, at all ages and in all forms of obesity. Unless this is so, we are entitled to harbor grave doubts as to whether a given treatment corrects the underlying disorder. Moreover, any claim that the disorder has been corrected must be substantiated by the ability of the patient to eat normally of any food he pleases without regaining abnormal fat after treatment. Only if these conditions are fulfilled can we legitimately speak of curing obesity rather than of reducing weight.

Our problem thus presents itself as an enquiry into the localization and the nature of the disorder which leads to obesity. The history of this enquiry is a long series of high hopes and bitter disappointments.

The History of Obesity
There was a time, not so long ago, when obesity was considered a sign of health and prosperity in man and of beauty, amorousness and fecundity in women. This attitude probably dates back to Neolithic times, about 8000 years ago; when for the first time in the history of culture, man began to own property, domestic animals, arable land, houses, pottery and metal tools. Before that, with the possible exception of some races such as the Hottentots, obesity was almost non-existent, as it still is in all wild animals and most primitive races.

Today obesity is extremely common among all civilized races, because a disposition to the disorder can be inherited. Wherever abnormal fat was regarded as an asset, sexual selection tended to propagate the trait. It is only in very recent times that manifest obesity has lost some of its allure, though the cult of the outsize bust – always a sign of latent obesity – shows that the trend still lingers on.

The Significance of Regular Meals
In the early Neolithic times another change took place which may well account for the fact that today nearly all inherited dispositions sooner or later develop into manifest obesity. This

change was the institution of regular meals. In pre-Neolithic times, man ate only when he was hungry and only as much as he required to still the pangs of hunger. Moreover, much of his food was raw and all of it was unrefined. He roasted his meat, but he did not boil it, as he had no pots, and what little he may have grubbed from the Earth and picked from the trees, he ate as he went along.

The whole structure of man's omnivorous digestive tract is, like that of an ape, rat or pig, adjusted to the continual nibbling of tidbits. It is not suited to occasional gorging as is, for instance, the intestine of the carnivorous cat family. Thus the institution of regular meals, particularly of food rendered rapidly assimilable, placed a great burden on modern man's ability to cope with large quantities of food suddenly pouring into his system from the intestinal tract.

The institution of regular meals meant that man had to eat more than his body required at the moment of eating so as to tide him over until the next meal. Food rendered easily digestible suddenly flooded his body with nourishment of which he was in no need at the moment. Somehow, somewhere this surplus had to be stored.

Three Kinds of Fat

In the human body we can distinguish three kinds of fat. The first is the structural fat which fills the gaps between various organs, a sort of packing material. Structural fat also performs such important functions as bedding the kidneys in soft elastic tissue, protecting the coronary arteries and keeping the skin smooth and taut. It also provides the springy cushion of hard fat under the bones of the feet, without which we would be unable to walk.

The second type of fat is a normal reserve of fuel upon which the body can freely draw when the nutritional income from the intestinal tract is insufficient to meet the demand. Such normal reserves are localized all over the body. Fat is a substance which packs the highest caloric value into the smallest space so that normal reserves of fuel for muscular activity and the maintenance of body temperature can be most economically stored in this form. Both these types of fat, structural and reserve, are normal, and even if the body stocks them to capacity this can never be called obesity.

But there is a third type of fat which is entirely abnormal. It is the accumulation of such fat, and of such fat only, from which the overweight patient suffers. This abnormal fat is also a potential reserve of fuel, but unlike the normal reserves it is not available to the body in a nutritional emergency. It is, so to speak, locked away in a fixed deposit and is not kept in a current account[2], as are the normal reserves.

When an obese patient tries to reduce by starving himself, he will first lose his normal fat reserves. When these are exhausted he begins to burn up structural fat, and only as a last resort will the body yield its abnormal reserves, though by that time the patient usually feels so weak and hungry that the diet is abandoned. It is just for this reason that obese patients complain that when they diet they lose the wrong fat. They feel famished and tired and their face becomes drawn and haggard, but their belly, hips, thighs and upper arms show little improvement. The fat they have come to detest stays on and the fat they need to cover their bones gets less and less. Their skin wrinkles and they look old and miserable. And that is one of the most frustrating and depressing experiences a human being can have.

Injustice to the Obese

When then obese patients are accused of cheating, gluttony, lack of will power, greed and sexual complexes, the strong become indignant and decide that modern medicine is a fraud and its representatives fools, while the weak just give up the struggle in despair. In either case the result is the same: a further gain in weight, resignation to an abominable fate and the resolution at least to live tolerably the short span allotted to them – a fig for doctors and insurance companies.

Obese patients only feel physically well as long as they are stationary or gaining weight. They may feel guilty, owing to the lethargy and indolence always associated with obesity. They may feel ashamed of what they have been led to believe is a lack of control. They may feel horrified by the appearance of their nude body and the tightness of their clothes. But they have a primitive feeling of animal content which turns to misery and suffering as soon as they make a resolute attempt to reduce. For this there are sound reasons.

In the first place, more caloric energy is required to keep a large body at a certain temperature than to heat a small body. Secondly the muscular effort of moving a heavy body is greater than in the case of a light body. The muscular effort consumes Calories which must be provided by food. Thus, all other factors being equal, a fat person requires more food than a lean one. One might therefore

---

[2] "Current account" is the British name for what Americans call a checking account.

reason that if a fat person eats only the additional food his body requires he should be able to keep his weight stationary. Yet every physician who has studied obese patients under rigorously controlled conditions knows that this is not true. Many obese patients actually gain weight on a diet which is calorically deficient for their basic needs. There must thus be some other mechanism at work

Glandular Theories

At one time it was thought that this mechanism might be concerned with the sex glands. Such a connection was suggested by the fact that many juvenile obese patients show an under-development of the sex organs. The middle-age spread in men and the tendency of many women to put on weight in the menopause seemed to indicate a causal connection between diminishing sex function and overweight. Yet, when highly active sex hormones became available, it was found that their administration had no effect whatsoever on obesity. The sex glands could therefore not be the seat of the disorder.

The Thyroid Gland

When it was discovered that the thyroid gland controls the rate at which body-fuel is consumed, it was thought that by administering thyroid gland to obese patients their abnormal fat deposits could be burned up more rapidly. This too proved to be entirely disappointing, because as we now know, these abnormal deposits take no part in the body's energy-turnover – they are inaccessibly locked away. Thyroid medication merely forces the body to consume its normal fat reserves, which are already depleted in obese patients, and then to break down structurally essential fat without touching the abnormal deposits. In this way a patient may be brought to the brink of starvation in spite of having a hundred pounds of fat to spare. Thus any weight loss brought about by thyroid medication is always at the expense of fat of which the body is in dire need.

While the majority of obese patients have a perfectly normal thyroid gland and some even have an overactive thyroid, one also occasionally sees a case with a real thyroid deficiency. In such cases, treatment with thyroid brings about a small loss of weight, but this is not due to the loss of any abnormal fat. It is entirely the result of the elimination of a mucoid substance, called myxedema, which the body accumulates when there is a marked primary thyroid deficiency. Moreover, patients suffering only from a severe lack of thyroid hormone never become obese in the true sense. Possibly also the
20

observation that normal persons – though not the obese – lose weight rapidly when their thyroid becomes overactive may have contributed to the false notion that thyroid deficiency and obesity are connected. Much misunderstanding about the supposed role of the thyroid gland in obesity is still met with, and it is now really high time that thyroid preparations be once and for all struck off the list of remedies for obesity. This is particularly so because giving thyroid gland to an obese patient whose thyroid is either normal or overactive, besides being useless, is decidedly dangerous.

The Pituitary Gland

The next gland to be falsely incriminated was the anterior lobe of the pituitary, or hypophysis. This most important gland lies well protected in a bony capsule at the base of the skull. It has a vast number of functions in the body, among which is the regulation of all the other important endocrine glands. The fact that various signs of anterior pituitary deficiency are often associated with obesity raised the hope that the seat of the disorder might be in this gland. But although a large number of pituitary hormones have been isolated and many extracts of the gland prepared, not a single one or any combination of such factors proved to be of any value in the treatment of obesity. Quite recently, however, a fat-mobilizing factor has been found in pituitary glands, but it is still too early to say whether this factor is destined to play a role in the treatment of obesity.

The Adrenals

Recently, a long series of brilliant discoveries concerning the working of the adrenal or suprarenal glands, small bodies which sit atop the kidneys, have created tremendous interest. This interest also turned to the problem of obesity when it was discovered that a condition which in some respects resembles a severe case of obesity – the so called Cushing's Syndrome – was caused by a glandular new-growth of the adrenals or by their excessive stimulation with ACTH, which is the pituitary hormone governing the activity of the outer rind or cortex of the adrenals.

When we learned that an abnormal stimulation of the adrenal cortex could produce signs that resemble true obesity, this knowledge furnished no practical means of treating obesity by decreasing the activity of the adrenal cortex. There is no evidence to suggest that in obesity there is any excess of adrenocortical activity; in fact, all the evidence points to the contrary. There seems to be rather a lack of adrenocortical function and a decrease in the secretion of ACTH from the anterior pituitary lobe.[3]

So here again our search for the mechanism which produces obesity led us into a blind alley. Recently, many students of obesity have reverted to the nihilistic attitude that obesity is caused simply by overeating and that it can only be cured by under eating.

The Diencephalon or Hypothalamus

For those of us who refused to be discouraged there remained one slight hope. Buried deep down in the massive human brain there is a part which we have in common with all vertebrate animals the so-called diencephalon. It is a very primitive part of the brain and has in man been almost smothered by the huge masses of nervous tissue with which we think, reason and voluntarily move our body. The diencephalon is the part from which the central nervous system controls all the automatic animal functions of the body, such as breathing, the heart beat, digestion, sleep, sex, the urinary system, the autonomous or vegetative nervous system and via the pituitary the whole interplay of the endocrine glands.

It was therefore not unreasonable to suppose that the complex operation of storing and issuing fuel to the body might also be controlled by the diencephalon. It has long been known that the content of sugar – another form of fuel – in the blood depends on a certain nervous center in the diencephalon. When this center is destroyed in laboratory animals, they develop a condition rather similar to human stable diabetes. It has also long been known that the destruction of another diencephalic center produces a voracious appetite and a rapid gain in weight in animals which never get fat spontaneously.

The Fat-bank

Assuming that in man such a center controlling the movement of fat does exist, its function would have to be much like that of a bank. When the body assimilates from the intestinal tract more fuel than it needs at the moment, this surplus is deposited in what may be

---

[3] There is some clinical evidence to suggest that those symptoms of Cushing's Syndrome which resemble true obesity are caused by the same mechanism which causes common obesity, while the other symptoms of the syndrome are directly due to adrenocortical dysfunction.

compared with a current account. Out of this account it can always be withdrawn as required. All normal fat reserves are in such a current account, and it is probable that a diencephalic center manages the deposits and withdrawals.

When now, for reasons which will be discussed later, the deposits grow rapidly while small withdrawals become more frequent, a point may be reached which goes beyond the diencephalon's banking capacity. Just as a banker might suggest to a wealthy client that instead of accumulating a large and unmanageable current account he should invest his surplus capital, the body appears to establish a fixed deposit into which all surplus funds go but from which they can no longer be withdrawn by the procedure used in a current account. In this way the diencephalic "fat-bank" frees itself from all work which goes beyond its normal banking capacity. The onset of obesity dates from the moment the diencephalon adopts this labor-saving ruse. Once a fixed deposit has been established the normal fat reserves are held at a minimum, while every available surplus is locked away in the fixed deposit and is therefore taken out of normal circulation.

THREE BASIC CAUSES OF OBESITY:

(1) The Inherited Factor

Assuming that there is a limit to the diencephalon's fat banking capacity, it follows that there are three basic ways in which obesity can become manifest. The first is that the fat-banking capacity is abnormally low from birth. Such a congenitally low diencephalic capacity would then represent the inherited factor in obesity. When this abnormal trait is markedly present, obesity will develop at an early age in spite of normal feeding; this could explain why among brothers and sisters eating the same food at the same table some become obese and others do not.

(2) Other Diencephalic Disorders

The second way in which obesity can become established is the lowering of a previously normal fat-banking capacity owing to some other diencephalic disorder. It seems to be a general rule that when one of the many diencephalic centers is particularly overtaxed; it tries to increase its capacity at the expense of other centers.

In the menopause and after castration the hormones previously produced in the sex-glands no longer circulate in the body. In the presence of normally functioning sex-glands their hormones act as a brake on the secretion of the sex-gland stimulating hormones of the anterior pituitary. When this brake is removed the anterior pituitary enormously increases its output of these sex-gland stimulating hormones, though they are now no longer effective. In the absence of any response from the non-functioning or missing sex glands, there is nothing to stop the anterior pituitary from producing more and more of these hormones. This situation causes an excessive strain on the diencephalic center which controls the function of the anterior pituitary. In order to cope with this additional burden the center appears to draw more and more energy away from other centers, such as those concerned with emotional stability, the blood circulation (hot flushes) and other autonomous nervous regulations, particularly also from the not so vitally important fat-bank.

The so-called stable type of diabetes heavily involves the diencephalic blood sugar regulating center. The diencephalon tries to meet this abnormal load by switching energy destined for the fat bank over to the sugar-regulating center, with the result that the fat-banking capacity is reduced to the point at which it is forced to establish a fixed deposit and thus initiate the disorder we call obesity. In this case one would have to consider the diabetes the primary cause of the obesity, but it is also possible that the process is reversed in the sense that a deficient or overworked fat-center draws energy from the sugar-center, in which case the obesity would be the cause of that type of diabetes in which the pancreas is not primarily involved. Finally, it is conceivable that in Cushing's syndrome those symptoms which resemble obesity are entirely due to the withdrawal of energy from the diencephalic fat-bank in order to make it available to the highly disturbed center which governs the anterior pituitary adrenocortical system.

Whether obesity is caused by a marked inherited deficiency of the fat-center or by some entirely different diencephalic regulatory disorder, its insurgence obviously has nothing to do with overeating and in either case obesity is certain to develop regardless of dietary restrictions. In these cases any enforced food deficit is made up from essential fat reserves and normal structural fat, much to the disadvantage of the patient's general health.

(3) The Exhaustion of the Fat-bank

But there is still a third way in which obesity can become established, and that is when a presumably normal fat-center is suddenly — the emphasis is on suddenly — called upon to deal with an enormous influx of food far in excess of momentary requirements. At first glance it does seem that here we have a straight-forward case of overeating being responsible for obesity, but on further analysis it soon becomes clear that the relation of cause and effect is not so simple. In the first place we are merely assuming that the capacity of the fat center is normal while it is possible and even probable that only persons who have some inherited trait in this direction can become obese merely by overeating.

Secondly, in many of these cases the amount of food eaten remains the same and it is only the consumption of fuel which is suddenly decreased, as when an athlete is confined to bed for many weeks with a broken bone or when a man leading a highly active life is suddenly tied to his desk in an office and to television at home. Similarly, when a person, grown up in a cold climate, is transferred to a tropical country and continues to eat as before, he may develop obesity because in the heat far less fuel is required to maintain the normal body temperature.

When a person suffers a long period of privation, be it due to chronic illness, poverty, famine or the exigencies of war, his diencephalic regulations adjust themselves to some extent to the low food intake. When then suddenly these conditions change and he is free to eat all the food he wants, this is liable to overwhelm his fat-regulating center. During the last war[4] about 6000 grossly underfed Polish refugees who had spent harrowing years in Russia were transferred to a camp in India where they were well housed, given normal British army rations and some cash to buy a few extras. Within about three months, 85% were suffering from obesity.

In a person eating coarse and unrefined food, the digestion is slow and only a little nourishment at a time is assimilated from the intestinal tract. When such a person is suddenly able to obtain highly refined foods such as sugar, white flour, butter and oil these are so rapidly digested and assimilated that the rush of incoming fuel which occurs at every meal may eventually overpower the diecenphalic regulatory mechanisms and thus lead to obesity. This is commonly

_____

[4] World War II.

seen in the poor man who suddenly becomes rich enough to buy the more expensive refined foods, though his total caloric intake remains the same or is even less than before.

Psychological Aspects

Much has been written about the psychological aspects of obesity. Among its many functions the diencephalon is also the seat of our primitive animal instincts, and just as in an emergency it can switch energy from one center to another, so it seems to be able to transfer pressure from one instinct to another. Thus, a lonely and unhappy person deprived of all emotional comfort and of all instinct gratification except the stilling of hunger and thirst can use these as outlets for pent up instinct pressure and so develop obesity. Yet once that has happened, no amount of psychotherapy or analysis, happiness, company or the gratification of other instincts will correct the condition.

Compulsive Eating

No end of injustice is done to obese patients by accusing them of compulsive eating, which is a form of diverted sex gratification. Most obese patients do not suffer from compulsive eating; they suffer genuine hunger – real, gnawing, torturing hunger – which has nothing whatever to do with compulsive eating. Even their sudden desire for sweets is merely the result of the experience that sweets, pastries and alcohol will most rapidly of all foods allay the pangs of hunger. This has nothing to do with diverted instincts.

On the other hand, compulsive eating does occur in some obese patients, particularly in girls in their late teens or early twenties. Compulsive eating differs fundamentally from the obese patient's greater need for food. It comes on in attacks and is never associated with real hunger, a fact which is readily admitted by the patients. They only feel a feral desire to stuff. Two pounds of chocolates may be devoured in a few minutes; cold, greasy food from the refrigerator, stale bread, leftovers on stacked plates, almost anything edible is crammed down with terrifying speed and ferocity.

I have occasionally been able to watch such an attack without the patient's knowledge, and it is a frightening, ugly spectacle to behold, even if one does realize that mechanisms entirely beyond the patient's control are at work. A careful enquiry into what may have brought on such an attack almost invariably reveals that it is preceded by a strong unresolved sex-stimulation, the higher centers of the brain having blocked primitive diencephalic instinct gratification. The pressure is then let off through another primitive channel, which is oral gratification. In my experience the only thing that will cure this condition is uninhibited sex, a therapeutic procedure which is hardly ever feasible, for if it were, the patient would have adopted it without professional prompting, nor would this in any way correct the associated obesity. It would only raise new and often greater problems if used as a therapeutic measure.

Patients suffering from real compulsive eating are comparatively rare. In my practice they constitute about 1-2%. Treating them for obesity is a heartrending job. They do perfectly well between attacks, but a single bout occurring while under treatment may annul several weeks of therapy. Little wonder that such patients become discouraged. In these cases I have found that psychotherapy may make the patient fully understand the mechanism, but it does nothing to stop it. Perhaps society's growing sexual permissiveness will make compulsive eating even rarer.

Whether a patient is really suffering from compulsive eating or not is hard to decide before treatment because many obese patients think that their desire for food — to them unmotivated — is due to compulsive eating, while all the time it is merely a greater need for food. The only way to find out is to treat such patients. Those that suffer from real compulsive eating continue to have such attacks, while those who are not compulsive eaters never get an attack during treatment.

Reluctance to Lose Weight

Some patients are deeply attached to their fat and cannot bear the thought of losing it. If they are intelligent, popular and successful in spite of their handicap, this is a source of pride. Some fat girls look upon their condition as a safeguard against erotic involvements, of which they are afraid. They work out a pattern of life in which their obesity plays a determining role and then become reluctant to upset this pattern and face a new kind of life which will be entirely different after their figure has become normal and often very attractive. They fear that people will like them – or be jealous – on account of their figure rather than be attracted by their intelligence or character only. Some have a feeling that reducing means giving up an almost cherished and intimate part of themselves. In many of these cases psychotherapy can be helpful, as it enables these patients to see the whole situation in the full light of consciousness. An affectionate attachment to abnormal fat is usually seen in patients who became obese in childhood, but this is not necessarily so.

In all other cases the best psychotherapy can do in the usual treatment of obesity is to render the burden of hunger and never-ending dietary restrictions slightly more tolerable. Patients who have successfully established an erotic transfer to their psychiatrist are often better able to bear their suffering as a secret labor of love.

There are thus a large number of ways in which obesity can be initiated, though the disorder itself is always due to the same mechanism, an inadequacy of the diencephalic fat-center and the laying down of abnormally fixed fat deposits in abnormal places. This means that once obesity has become established, it can no more be cured by eliminating those factors which brought it on than a fire can be extinguished by removing the cause of the conflagration. Thus a discussion of the various ways in which obesity can become established is useful from a preventative point of view, but it has no bearing on the treatment of the established condition. The elimination of factors which are clearly hastening the course of the disorder may slow down its progress or even halt it, but they can never correct it.

Not by Weight Alone…

Weight alone is not a satisfactory criterion by which to judge whether a person is suffering from the disorder we call obesity or not. Every physician is familiar with the sylphlike lady who enters the consulting room and declares emphatically that she is getting horribly fat and wishes to reduce. Many an honest and sympathetic physician at once concludes that he is dealing with a "nut." If he is busy he will give her short shrift, but if he has time he will weigh her and show her tables to prove that she is actually underweight.

I have never yet seen or heard of such a lady being convinced by either procedure. The reason is that in my experience the lady is nearly always right and the doctor wrong. When such a patient is carefully examined one finds many signs of potential obesity, which is just about to become manifest as overweight. The patient distinctly feels that something is wrong with her, that a subtle change is taking place in her body, and this alarms her.

There are a number of signs and symptoms which are characteristic of obesity. In manifest obesity many and often all these signs and symptoms are present. In latent or just beginning cases some are always found, and it should be a rule that if two or more of the bodily signs are present, the case must be regarded as one that needs immediate help.

28

Signs and Symptoms of Obesity

The bodily signs may be divided into such as have developed before puberty, indicating a strong inherited factor, and those which develop at the onset of manifest disorder. Early signs are a disproportionately large size of the two upper front teeth, the first incisor, or a dimple on both sides of the sacral bone just above the buttocks. When the arms are outstretched with the palms upward, the forearms appear sharply angled outward from the upper arms. The same applies to the lower extremities. The patient cannot bring his feet together without the knees overlapping; he is, in fact, knock-kneed.

The beginning accumulation of abnormal fat shows as a little pad just below the nape of the neck, colloquially known as the Duchess' Hump. There is a triangular fatty bulge in front of the armpit when the arm is held against the body. When the skin is stretched by fat rapidly accumulating under it, it may split in the lower layers. When large and fresh, such tears are purple, but later they are transformed into white scar-tissue. Such striation, as it is called, commonly occurs on the abdomen of women during pregnancy, but in obesity it is frequently found on the breasts, the hips and occasionally on the shoulders. In many cases striation is so fine that the small white lines are only just visible. They are always a sure sign of obesity, and though this may be slight at the time of examination such patients can usually remember a period in their childhood when they were excessively chubby.

Another typical sign is a pad of fat on the insides of the knees, a spot where normal fat reserves are never stored. There may be a fold of skin over the pubic area and another fold may stretch round both sides of the chest, where a loose roll of fat can be picked up between two fingers. In the male an excessive accumulation of fat in the breasts is always indicative, while in the female the breast is usually, but not necessarily, large. Obviously excessive fat on the abdomen, the hips, thighs, upper arms, chin and shoulders are characteristic, and it is important to remember that any number of these signs may be present in persons whose weight is statistically normal; particularly if they are dieting on their own with iron determination.

Common clinical symptoms which are indicative only in their association and in the frame of the whole clinical picture are: frequent headaches, rheumatic pains without detectable bony abnormality; a feeling of laziness and lethargy, often both physical and mental and

29

frequently associated with insomnia, the patients saying that all they want is to rest; the frightening feeling of being famished and sometimes weak with hunger two to three hours after a hearty meal and an irresistible yearning for sweets and starchy food which often overcomes the patient quite suddenly and is sometimes substituted by a desire for alcohol; constipation and a spastic or irritable colon are unusually common among the obese, and so are menstrual disorders.

Returning once more to our sylphlike lady, we can say that a combination of some of these symptoms with a few of the typical bodily signs is sufficient evidence to take her case seriously. A human figure, male or female, can only be judged in the nude; any opinion based on the dressed appearance can be quite fantastically wide off the mark, and I feel myself driven to the conclusion that apart from frankly psychotic patients such as cases of anorexia nervosa; a morbid weight fixation does not exist. I have yet to see a patient who continues to complain after the figure has been rendered normal by adequate treatment.

The Emaciated Lady

I remember the case of a lady who was escorted into my consulting room while I was telephoning. She sat down in front of my desk, and when I looked up to greet her I saw the typical picture of advanced emaciation. Her dry skin hung loosely over the bones of her face, her neck was scrawny and collarbones and ribs stuck out from deep hollows. I immediately thought of cancer and decided to which of my colleagues at the hospital I would refer her. Indeed, I felt a little annoyed that my assistant had not explained to her that her case did not fall under my specialty. In answer to my query as to what I could do for her, she replied that she wanted to reduce. I tried to hide my surprise, but she must have noted a fleeting expression, for she smiled and said "I know that you think I'm mad, but just wait." With that she rose and came round to my side of the desk. Jutting out from a tiny waist she had enormous hips and thighs.

By using a technique which will presently be described, the abnormal fat on her hips was transferred to the rest of her body which had been emaciated by months of very severe dieting. At the end of a treatment lasting five weeks, she, a small woman, had lost 8 inches round her hips, while her face looked fresh and florid, the ribs were no longer visible and her weight was the same to the ounce as it had been at the first consultation.

Fat but Not Obese

While a person who is statistically underweight may still be suffering from the disorder which causes obesity, it is also possible for a person to be statistically overweight without suffering from obesity. For such persons weight is no problem, as they can gain or lose at will and experience no difficulty in reducing their caloric intake. They are masters of their weight, which the obese are not. Moreover, their excess fat shows no preference for certain typical regions of the body, as does the fat in all cases of obesity. Thus, the decision whether a borderline case is really suffering from obesity or not cannot be made merely by consulting weight tables.

THE TREATMENT OF OBESITY

If obesity is always due to one very specific diencephalic deficiency, it follows that the only way to cure it is to correct this deficiency. At first this seemed an utterly hopeless undertaking. The greatest obstacle was that one could hardly hope to correct an inherited trait localized deep inside the brain, and while we did possess a number of drugs whose point of action was believed to be in the diencephalon, none of them had the slightest effect on the fat-center. There was not even a pointer showing a direction in which pharmacological research could move to find a drug that had such a specific action. The closest approach were the appetite-reducing drugs – the amphetamines----- but these cured nothing.

Curious Observation

Mulling over this depressing situation, I remembered a rather curious observation made many years ago in India. At that time we knew very little about the function of the diencephalon, and my interest centered round the pituitary gland. Froehlich had described cases of extreme obesity and sexual underdevelopment in youths suffering from a new growth of the anterior pituitary lobe, producing what then became known as Froehlich's disease. However, it was very soon discovered that the identical syndrome, though running a less fulminating course, was quite common in patients whose pituitary gland was perfectly normal. These are the so-called "fat boys" with long, slender hands, breasts any flat-chested maiden would be proud to possess, large hips, buttocks and thighs with striation, knock-knees and underdeveloped genitals, often with undescended testicles.

It also became known that in these cases the sex organs could he developed by giving the patients injections of a substance extracted from the urine of pregnant women, it having been shown that when this substance was injected into sexually immature rats it made them precociously mature. The amount of substance which produced this effect in one rat was called one International Unit, and the purified extract was accordingly called "Human Chorionic Gonadotrophin" whereby chorionic signifies that it is produced in the placenta and gonadotropin that its action is sex gland directed.

The usual way of treating "fat boys" with underdeveloped genitals is to inject several hundred International Units twice a week. Human Chorionic Gonadotrophin which we shall henceforth simply call HCG is expensive and as "fat boys" are fairly common among Indians I tried to establish the smallest effective dose. In the course of this study three interesting things emerged. The first was that when fresh pregnancy-urine from the female ward was given in quantities of about 300 cc. by retention enema, as good results could be obtained as by injecting the pure substance. The second was that small daily doses appeared to be just as effective as much larger ones given twice a week. Thirdly, and that is the observation that concerns us here, when such patients were given small daily doses they seemed to lose their ravenous appetite though they neither gained nor lost weight. Strangely enough however, their shape did change. Though they were not restricted in diet, there was a distinct decrease in the circumference of their hips.

Fat on the Move

Remembering this, it occurred to me that the change in shape could only be explained by a movement of fat away from abnormal deposits on the hips, and if that were so there was just a chance that while such fat was in transition it might be available to the body as fuel. This was easy to find out, as in that case, fat on the move would be able to replace food. It should then he possible to keep a "fat boy" on a severely restricted diet without a feeling of hunger, in spite of a rapid loss of weight. When I tried this in typical cases of Froehlich's syndrome, I found that as long as such patients were given small daily doses of HCG they could comfortably go about their usual occupations on a diet of only 500 Calories daily and lose an average of about one pound per day. It was also perfectly evident that only abnormal fat was being consumed, as there were no signs of any depletion of normal fat. Their skin remained fresh and turgid, and gradually their figures became entirely normal, nor did the daily
32

administration of HCG appear to have any side-effects other than beneficial.

From this point it was a small step to try the same method in all other forms of obesity. It took a few hundred cases to establish beyond reasonable doubt that the mechanism operates in exactly the same way and seemingly without exception in every case of obesity. I found that, though most patients were treated in the outpatients department, gross dietary errors rarely occurred. On the contrary, most patients complained that the two meals of 250 Calories each were more than they could manage, as they continually had a feeling of just having had a large meal.

Pregnancy and Obesity

Once this trail was opened, further observations seemed to fall into line. It is, for instance, well known that during pregnancy an obese woman can very easily lose weight. She can drastically reduce her diet without feeling hunger or discomfort and lose weight without in any way harming the child in her womb. It is also surprising to what extent a woman can suffer from pregnancy-vomiting without coming to any real harm.

Pregnancy is an obese woman's one great chance to reduce her excess weight. That she so rarely makes use of this opportunity is due to the erroneous notion, usually fostered by her elder relations, that she now has "two mouths to feed" and must "keep up her strength for the coming event." All modern obstetricians know that this is nonsense and that the more superfluous fat is lost the less difficult will be the confinement, though some still hesitate to prescribe a diet sufficiently low in Calories to bring about a drastic reduction.

A woman may gain weight during pregnancy, but she never becomes obese in the strict sense of the word. Under the influence of the HCG which circulates in enormous quantities in her body during pregnancy, her diencephalic banking capacity seems to be unlimited, and abnormal fixed deposits are never formed. At confinement[5] she is suddenly deprived of HCG, and her diencephalic fat-center reverts to its normal capacity. It is only then that the abnormally accumulated fat is locked away again in a fixed deposit. From that moment on she is suffering from obesity and is subject to all its consequences.

---

[5] Confinement = the concluding state of pregnancy

Pregnancy seems to be the only normal human condition in which the diencephalic fat-banking capacity is unlimited. It is only during pregnancy that fixed fat deposits can be transferred back into the normal current account and freely drawn upon to make up for any nutritional deficit. During pregnancy, every ounce of reserve fat is placed at the disposal of the growing fetus. Were this not so, an obese woman, whose normal reserves are already depleted, would have the greatest difficulties in bringing her pregnancy to full term. There is considerable evidence to suggest that it is the HCG produced in large quantities in the placenta which brings about this diencephalic change.

Though we may be able to increase the dieneephalic fat banking capacity by injecting HCG, this does not in itself affect the weight, just as transferring monetary funds from a fixed deposit into a current account does not make a man any poorer; to become poorer it is also necessary that he freely spends the money which thus becomes available. In pregnancy the needs of the growing embryo take care of this to some extent, but in the treatment of obesity there is no embryo, and so a very severe dietary restriction must take its place for the duration of treatment.

Only when the fat which is in transit under the effect of HCG is actually consumed can more fat be withdrawn from the fixed deposits. In pregnancy it would be most undesirable if the fetus were offered ample food only when there is a high influx from the intestinal tract. Ideal nutritional conditions for the fetus can only be achieved when the mother's blood is continually saturated with food, regardless of whether she eats or not, as otherwise a period of starvation might hamper the steady growth of the embryo. It seems that HCG brings about this continual saturation of the blood, which is the reason why obese patients under treatment with HCG never feel hungry in spite of their drastically reduced food intake.

The Nature of Human Chorionic Gonadotrophin

HCG is never found in the human body except during pregnancy and in those rare cases in which a residue of placental tissue continues to grow in the womb in what is known as a chorionic epithelioma. It is never found in the male. The human type of chorionic gonadotrophin is found only during the pregnancy of women and the great apes. It is produced in enormous quantities, so that during certain phases of her pregnancy a woman may excrete as much as one million International Units per day in her urine – enough to render a million infantile rats precociously mature. Other mammals

34

make use of a different hormone, which can be extracted from their blood serum but not from their urine. Their placenta differs in this and other respects from that of man and the great apes. This animal chorionic gonadotrophin is much less rapidly broken down in the human body than HCG, and it is also less suitable for the treatment of obesity.

As often happens in medicine, much confusion has been caused by giving HCG its name before its true mode of action was understood. It has been explained that gonadotrophin literally means a sex-gland directed substance or hormone, and this is quite misleading. It dates from the early days when it was first found that HCG is able to render infantile sex glands mature, whereby it was entirely overlooked that it has no stimulating effect whatsoever on normally developed and normally functioning sex-glands. No amount of HCG is ever able to increase a normal sex function; it can only improve an abnormal one and in the young hasten the onset of puberty. However, this is no direct effect. HCG acts exclusively at a diencephalic level and there brings about a considerable increase in the functional capacity of all those centers which are working at maximum capacity.

The Real Gonadotrophins

Two hormones known in the female as follicle stimulating hormone (FSH) and corpus luteum stimulating hormone (LSH) are secreted by the anterior lobe of the pituitary gland. These hormones are real gonadotrophins because they directly govern the function of the ovaries. The anterior pituitary is in turn governed by the diencephalon, and so when there is an ovarian deficiency the diencephalic center concerned is hard put to correct matters by increasing the secretion from the anterior pituitary of FSH or LSH, as the case may be. When sexual deficiency is clinically present, this is a sign that the diencephalic center concerned is unable, in spite of maximal exertion, to cope with the demand for anterior pituitary stimulation.[6] When then the administration of HCG increases the functional capacity of the diencephalon, all demands can be fully satisfied and the sex deficiency is corrected.

----

[6] As we are speaking of purely regulatory disorders, we obviously exclude all such cases in which there are gross organic lesions of the pituitary or of the sex-glands themselves.

That this is the true mechanism underlying the presumed gonadotrophic action of HCG is confirmed by the fact that when the pituitary gland of infantile rats is removed before they are given HCG, the latter has no effect on their sex-glands. HCG cannot therefore have a direct sex gland stimulating action like that of the anterior pituitary gonadotrophins, as FSH and LSH are justly called. The latter are entirely different substances from that which can be extracted from pregnancy urine and which, unfortunately, is called chorionic gonadotrophin. It would be no more clumsy, and certainly far more appropriate, if HCG were henceforth called chorionic diencephalotrophin.

HCG No Sex Hormone

It cannot he sufficiently emphasized that HCG is not sex-hormone, that its action is identical in men, women, children and in those cases in which the sex-glands no longer function owing to old age or their surgical removal. The only sexual change it can bring about after puberty is an improvement of a pre-existing deficiency, but never a stimulation beyond the normal. In an indirect way via the anterior pituitary, HCG regulates menstruation and facilitates conception, but it never virilizes a woman or feminizes a man. It neither makes men grow breasts nor does it interfere with their virility, though where this was deficient it may improve it. It never makes women grow a beard or develop a gruff voice. I have stressed this point only for the sake of my lay readers, because, it is our daily experience that when patients hear the word hormone they immediately jump to the conclusion that this must have something to do with the sex- sphere. They are not accustomed as we are, to think thyroid, insulin, cortisone, adrenalin etc, as hormones.

Importance and Potency of HCG

Owing to the fact that HCG has no direct action on any endocrine gland, its enormous importance in pregnancy has been overlooked and its potency underestimated. Though a pregnant woman can produce as much as one million units per day, we find that the injection of only 125 units per day is ample to reduce weight at the rate of roughly one pound per day, even in a colossus weighing 400 pounds, when associated with a 500-Calorie diet. It is no exaggeration to say that the flooding of the female body with HCG is by far the most spectacular hormonal event in pregnancy. It has an enormous protective importance for mother and child, and I even go

36

so far as to say that no woman, and certainly not an obese one, could carry her pregnancy to term without it.

If I can be forgiven for comparing my fellow-endocrinologists with wicked Godmothers, HCG has certainly been their Cinderella, and I can only romantically hope that its extraordinary effect on abnormal fat will prove to be its Fairy Godmother.

HCG has been known for over half a century. It is the substance which Aschheim and Zondek so brilliantly used to diagnose early pregnancy out of the urine. Apart from that, the only thing it did in the experimental laboratory was to produce precocious rats, and that was not particularly stimulating to further research at a time when much more thrilling endocrinological discoveries were pouring in from all sides, sweeping, HCG into the stiller back waters.

Complicating Disorders

Some complicating disorders are often associated with obesity, and these we must briefly discuss. The most important associated disorders and the ones in which obesity seems to play a precipitating or at least an aggravating role are the following: the stable type of diabetes, gout, rheumatism and arthritis, high blood pressure and hardening of the arteries, coronary disease and cerebral hemorrhage.

Apart from the fact that they are often – though not necessarily – associated with obesity, these disorders have two things in common. In all of them, modern research is becoming more and more inclined to believe that diencephalic regulations play a dominant role in their causation. The other common factor is that they either improve or do not occur during pregnancy. In the latter respect they are joined by many other disorders not necessarily associated with obesity. Such disorders are, for instance, colitis, duodenal or gastric ulcers, certain allergies, psoriasis, loss of hair, brittle fingernails, migraine, etc.

If HCG + diet does in the obese bring about those diencephalic changes which are characteristic of pregnancy, one would expect to see an improvement in all these conditions comparable to that seen in real pregnancy. The administration of HCG does in fact do this in a remarkable way.

Diabetes

In an obese patient suffering from a fairly advanced case of stable diabetes of many years duration in which the blood sugar may range from 3-400 mg%, it is often possible to stop all antidiabetic medication after the first few days of treatment. The blood sugar continues to drop from day to day and often reaches normal values in 2-3 weeks. As in pregnancy, this phenomenon is not observed in the brittle type of diabetes, and as some cases that are predominantly stable may have a small brittle factor in their clinical makeup, all obese diabetics have to be kept under a very careful and expert watch.

A brittle case of diabetes is primarily due to the inability of the pancreas to produce sufficient insulin, while in the stable type, diencephalic regulations seem to be of greater importance. That is possibly the reason why the stable form responds so well to the HCG method of treating obesity, whereas the brittle type does not. Obese patients are generally suffering from the stable type, but a stable type may gradually change into a brittle one, which is usually associated with a loss of weight. Thus, when an obese diabetic finds that he is losing weight without diet or treatment, he should at once have his diabetes expertly attended to. There is some evidence to suggest that the change from stable to brittle is more liable to occur in patients who are taking insulin for their stable diabetes.

Rheumatism

All rheumatic pains, even those associated with demonstrable bony lesions, improve subjectively within a few days of treatment, and often require neither cortisone nor salicylates. Again this is a well-known phenomenon in pregnancy, and while under treatment with HCG + diet the effect is no less dramatic. As it does after pregnancy, the pain of deformed joints returns after treatment, but smaller doses of pain-relieving drugs seem able to control it satisfactorily after weight reduction. In any case, the HCG method makes it possible in obese arthritic patients to interrupt prolonged cortisone treatment without a recurrence of pain. This in itself is most welcome, but there is the added advantage that the treatment stimulates the secretion of ACTH in a physiological manner and that this regenerates the adrenal cortex, which is apt to suffer under prolonged cortisone treatment.

38

Cholesterol

The exact extent to which the blood cholesterol is involved in hardening of the arteries, high blood pressure and coronary disease is not as yet known, but it is now widely admitted that the blood cholesterol level is governed by diencephalic mechanisms. The behavior of circulating cholesterol is therefore of particular interest during the treatment of obesity with HCG. Cholesterol circulates in two forms, which we call free and esterified. Normally these fractions are present in a proportion of about 25% free to 75% esterified cholesterol, and it is the latter fraction which damages the walls of the arteries. In pregnancy this proportion is reversed and it may be taken for granted that arteriosclerosis never gets worse during pregnancy for this very reason.

To my knowledge, the only other condition in which the proportion of free to esterified cholesterol is reversed is during the treatment of obesity with HCG + diet, when exactly the same phenomenon takes place. This seems an important indication of how closely a patient under HCG treatment resembles a pregnant woman in diencephalic behavior.

When the total amount of circulating cholesterol is normal before treatment, this absolute amount is neither significantly increased nor decreased. But when an obese patient with an abnormally high cholesterol and already showing signs of arteriosclerosis is treated with HCG, his blood pressure drops and his coronary circulation seems to improve, and yet his total blood cholesterol may soar to heights never before reached.

At first this greatly alarmed us. But then we saw that the patients came to no harm even if treatment was continued and we found in follow-up examinations undertaken some months after treatment that the cholesterol was much better than it had been before treatment. As the increase is mostly in the form of the not dangerous free cholesterol, we gradually came to welcome the phenomenon. Today we believe that the rise is entirely due to the liberation of recent cholesterol deposits that have not yet undergone calcification in the arterial wall and therefore highly beneficial.

Gout

An identical behavior is found in the blood uric acid level of patients suffering from gout. Predictably such patients get an acute and often severe attack after the first few days of HCG treatment but then remain entirely free of pain, in spite of the fact that their blood uric acid often shows a marked increase which may persist for several months after treatment. Those patients who have regained their normal weight remain free of symptoms regardless of what they eat, while those that require a second course of treatment get another attack of gout as soon as the second course is initiated. We do not yet know what diencephalic mechanisms are involved in gout; possibly emotional factors play a role, and it is worth remembering that the disease does not occur in women of childbearing age. We now give 2 tablets daily of ZYLORIC to all patients who give a history of gout and have a high blood uric acid level. In this way we can completely avoid attacks during treatment.

Blood Pressure

Patients who have brought themselves to the brink of malnutrition by exaggerated dieting, laxatives etc, often have an abnormally low blood pressure. In these cases the blood pressure rises to normal values at the beginning of treatment and then very gradually drops, as it always does in patients with a normal blood pressure. Normal values are always regained a few days after the treatment is over. Of this lowering of the blood pressure during treatment the patients are not aware. When the blood pressure is abnormally high, and provided there are no detectable renal lesions, the pressure drops, as it usually does in pregnancy. The drop is often very rapid, so rapid in fact that it sometimes is advisable to slow down the process with pressure sustaining medication until the circulation has had a few days' time to adjust itself to the new situation. On the other hand, among the thousands of cases treated, we have never seen any untoward incident which could be attributed to the rather sudden drop in high blood pressure.

When a woman suffering from high blood pressure becomes pregnant her blood pressure very soon drops, but after her confinement it may gradually rise back to its former level. Similarly, a high blood pressure present before HCG treatment tends to rise again after the treatment is over, though this is not always the case. But the former high levels are rarely reached, and we have gathered the impression that such relapses respond better to orthodox drugs such as Reserpine than before treatment.

Peptic Ulcers

In our cases of obesity with gastric or duodenal ulcers we have noticed a surprising subjective improvement in spite of a diet

40

which would generally be considered most inappropriate for an ulcer patient. Here, too, there is a similarity with pregnancy, in which peptic ulcers hardly ever occur. However we have seen two cases with a previous history of several hemorrhages in which a bleeding occurred within 2 weeks of the end of treatment.

Psoriasis, Fingernails, Hair, Varicose Ulcers

As in pregnancy, psoriasis greatly improves during treatment but may relapse when the treatment is over. Most patients spontaneously report a marked improvement in the condition of brittle fingernails. The loss of hair not infrequently associated with obesity is temporarily arrested, though in very rare cases an increased loss of hair has been reported. I remember a case in which a patient developed a patchy baldness – so called *alopecia areata* – after a severe emotional shock, just before she was about to start an HCG treatment. Our dermatologist diagnosed the case as a particularly severe one, predicting that all the hair would be lost. He counseled against the reducing treatment, but in view of my previous experience and as the patient was very anxious not to postpone reducing, I discussed the matter with the dermatologist and it was agreed that, having fully acquainted the patient with the situation, the treatment should be started. During the treatment, which lasted four weeks, the further development of the bald patches was almost, if not quite, arrested; however, within a week of having finished the course of HCG, all the remaining hair fell out as predicted by the dermatologist. The interesting point is that the treatment was able to postpone this result but not to prevent it. The patient has now grown a new shock of hair of which she is justly proud.

In obese patients with large varicose ulcers we were surprised to find that these ulcers heal rapidly under treatment with HCG. We have since treated non obese patients suffering from varicose ulcers with daily injections of HCG on normal diet with equally good results.

The "Pregnant" Male

When a male patient hears that he is about to be put into a condition which in some respects resembles pregnancy, he is usually shocked and horrified. The physician must therefore carefully explain that this does not mean that he will be feminized and that HCG in no way interferes with his sex. He must be made to understand that in the interest of the propagation of the species nature provides for a

41

perfect functioning of the regulatory headquarters in the diencephalon during pregnancy and that we are merely using this natural safeguard as a means of correcting the diencephalic disorder which is responsible for his overweight.

TECHNIQUE

Warnings

I must warn the lay reader that what follows is mainly for the treating physician and most certainly not a do-it-yourself primer. Many of the expressions used mean something entirely different to a qualified doctor than that which their common use implies, and only a physician can correctly interpret the symptoms which may arise during treatment. Any patient who thinks he can reduce by taking a few "shots" and eating less is not only sure to be disappointed but may be heading for serious trouble. The benefit the patient can derive from reading this part of the book is a fuller realization of how very important it is for him to follow to the letter his physician's instructions.

In treating obesity with the HCG + diet method we are handling what is perhaps the most complex organ in the human body. The diencephalon's functional equilibrium is delicately poised, so that whatever happens in one part has repercussions in others. In obesity this balance is out of kilter and can only be restored if the technique I am about to describe is followed implicitly. Even seemingly insignificant deviations, particularly those that at first sight seem to be an improvement, are very liable to produce most disappointing results and even annul the effect completely. For instance, if the diet is increased from 500 to 600 or 700 Calories, the loss of weight is quite unsatisfactory. If the daily dose of HCG is raised to 200 or more units daily its action often appears to be reversed, possibly because larger doses evoke diencephalic counter-regulations. On the other hand, the diencephalon is an extremely robust organ in spite of its unbelievable intricacy. From an evolutionary point of view it is one of the oldest organs in our body and its evolutionary history dates back more than 500 million years. This has tendered it extraordinarily adaptable to all natural exigencies, and that is one of the main reasons why the human species was able to evolve. What its evolution did not prepare it for were the conditions to which human culture and civilization now expose it.

History Taking

When a patient first presents himself for treatment, we take a general history and note the time when the first signs of overweight were observed. We try to establish the highest weight the patient has ever had in his life (obviously excluding pregnancy), when this was, and what measures have hitherto been taken in an effort to reduce.

It has been our experience that those patients who have been taking thyroid preparations for long periods have a slightly lower average loss of weight under treatment with HCG than those who have never taken thyroid. This is even so in those patients who have been taking thyroid because they had an abnormally low basal metabolic rate. In many of these cases the low BMR is not due to any intrinsic deficiency of the thyroid gland, but rather to a lack of diencephalic stimulation of the thyroid gland via the anterior pituitary lobe. We never allow thyroid to be taken during treatment, and yet a BMR which was very low before treatment is usually found to be normal after a week or two of HCG + diet. Needless to say, this does not apply to those cases in which a thyroid deficiency has been produced by the surgical removal of a part of an overactive gland. It is also most important to ascertain whether the patient has taken diuretics (water eliminating pills) as this also decreases the weight loss under the HCG regimen.

Returning to our procedure, we next ask the patient a few questions to which he is held to reply simply with "yes" or "no". These questions are: Do you suffer from headaches? rheumatic pains? menstrual disorders? constipation? breathlessness on exertion? swollen ankles? Do you consider yourself greedy? Do you feel the need to eat snacks between meals?

The patient then strips and is weighed and measured. The normal weight for his height, age, skeletal and muscular build is established from tables of statistical averages, whereby in women it is often necessary to make an allowance for particularly large and heavy breasts. The degree of overweight is then calculated, and from this the duration of treatment can be roughly assessed on the basis of an average loss of weight of a little less than a pound, say 300-400 grams-per injection, per day. It is a particularly interesting feature of the HCG treatment that in reasonably cooperative patients this figure is remarkably constant, regardless of sex, age and degree of overweight.

The Duration of Treatment

Patients who need to lose 15 pounds (7 kg.) or less require 26 days treatment with 23 daily injections. The extra three days are needed because all patients must continue the 500-Calorie diet for three days after the last injection. This is a very essential part of the treatment, because if they start eating normally as long as there is even a trace of HCG in their body they put on weight alarmingly at the end of the treatment. After three days when all the HCG has been eliminated this does not happen, because the blood is then no longer saturated with food and can thus accommodate an extra influx from the intestines without increasing its volume by retaining water.

We never give a treatment lasting less than 26 days, even in patients needing to lose only 5 pounds. It seems that even in the mildest cases of obesity the diencephalon requires about three weeks rest from the maximal exertion to which it has been previously subjected in order to regain fully its normal fat-banking capacity. Clinically this expresses itself, in the fact that, when in these mild cases, treatment is stopped as soon as the weight is normal, which may be achieved in a week, it is much more easily regained than after a full course of 23 injections.

As soon as such patients have lost all their abnormal superfluous fat, they at once begin to feel ravenously hungry in spite of continued injections. This is because HCG only puts abnormal fat into circulation and cannot, in the doses used, liberate normal fat deposits; indeed, it seems to prevent their consumption. As soon as their statistically normal weight is reached, these patients are put on 800-1000 Calories for the rest of the treatment. The diet is arranged in such a way that the weight remains perfectly stationary and is thus continued for three days after the 23rd injection. Only then are the patients free to eat anything they please except sugar and starches for the next three weeks.

Such early cases are common among actresses, models, and persons who are tired of obesity, having seen its ravages in other members of their family. Film actresses frequently explain that they must weigh less than normal. With this request we flatly refuse to comply, first, because we undertake to cure a disorder, not to create a new one, and second, because it is in the nature of the HCG method that it is self limiting. It becomes completely ineffective as soon as all abnormal fat is consumed. Actresses with a slight tendency to obesity, having tried all manner of reducing methods, invariably come to the conclusion that their figure is satisfactory only when they are underweight, simply because none of these methods remove their superfluous fat deposits. When they see that under HCG their figure improves out of all proportion to the amount of weight lost, they are nearly always content to remain within their normal weight-range.

When a patient has more than 15 pounds to lose the treatment takes longer but the maximum we give in a single course is 40 injections, nor do we as a rule allow patients to lose more than 34 lbs. (15 Kg.) at a time. The treatment is stopped when either 34 lbs. have been lost or 40 injections have been given. The only exception we make is in the case of grotesquely obese patients who may be allowed to lose an additional 5-6 lbs. if this occurs before the 40 injections are up.

Immunity to HCG

The reason for limiting a course to 40 injections is that by then some patients may begin to show signs of HCG immunity. Though this phenomenon is well known, we cannot as yet define the underlying mechanism. Maybe after a certain length of time the body learns to break down and eliminate HCG very rapidly, or possibly prolonged treatment leads to some sort of counter-regulation which annuls the diencephalic effect.

After 40 daily injections it takes about six weeks before this so called immunity is lost and HCG again becomes fully effective. Usually after about 40 injections patients may feel the onset of immunity as hunger which was previously absent. In those comparatively rare cases in which signs of immunity develop before the full course of 40 injections has been completed-say at the 35th injection- treatment must be stopped at once, because if it is continued the patients begin to look weary and drawn, feel weak and hungry and any further loss of weight achieved is then always at the expense of normal fat. This is not only undesirable, but normal fat is also instantly regained as soon as the patient is returned to a free diet.

Patients who need only 23 injections may be injected daily, including Sundays, as they never develop immunity. In those that take 40 injections the onset of immunity can be delayed if they are given only six injections a week, leaving out Sundays or any other day they choose, provided that it is always the same day. On the days on which they do not receive the injections they usually feel a slight sensation of hunger. At first we thought that this might be purely psychological, but we found that when normal saline is injected without the patient's knowledge the same phenomenon occurs.

Menstruation

During menstruation no injections are given, but the diet is continued and causes no hardship; yet as soon as the menstruation is over, the patients become extremely hungry unless the injections are resumed at once. It is very impressive to see the suffering of a woman who has continued her diet for a day or two beyond the end of the period without coming for her injection and then to hear the next day that all hunger ceased within a few hours after the injection and to see her once again content, florid and cheerful. While on the question of menstruation it must be added that in teenaged girls the period may in some rare cases be delayed and exceptionally stop altogether. If then later this is artificially induced some weight may be regained.

Further Courses

Patients requiring the loss of more than 34 lbs. must have a second or even more courses. A second course can be started after an interval of not less than six weeks, though the pause can be more than six weeks. When a third, fourth or even fifth course is necessary, the interval between courses should be made progressively longer. Between a second and third course eight weeks should elapse, between a third and fourth course twelve weeks, between a fourth and fifth course twenty weeks and between a fifth and sixth course six months. In this way it is possible to bring about a weight reduction of 100 lbs. and more if required without the least hardship to the patient.

In general, men do slightly better than women and often reach a somewhat higher average daily loss. Very advanced cases do a little better than early ones, but it is a remarkable fact that this difference is only just statistically significant.

Conditions That Must Be Accepted Before Treatment

On the basis of these data the probable duration of treatment can he calculated with considerable accuracy, and this is explained to the patient. It is made clear to him that during the course of treatment he must attend the clinic daily to be weighed, injected and generally checked. All patients that live in Rome or have resident friends or relations with whom they can stay are treated as out-patients, but patients coming from abroad must stay in the hospital, as no hotel or restaurant can be relied upon to prepare the diet with sufficient accuracy. These patients have their meals, sleep, and attend the clinic in the hospital, but are otherwise free to spend their time as they please in the city and its surroundings sightseeing, bathing or theater-going.

46

It is also made clear that between courses the patient gets no treatment and is free to eat anything he pleases except starches and sugar during the first 3 weeks. It is impressed upon him that he will have to follow the prescribed diet to the letter and that after the first three days this will cost him no effort, as he will feel no hunger and may indeed have difficulty in getting down the 500 Calories which he will be given. If these conditions are not acceptable the case is refused, as any compromise or half measure is bound to prove utterly disappointing to patient and physician alike and is a waste of time and energy.

Though a patient can only consider himself really cured when he has been reduced to his statistically normal weight, we do not insist that he commit himself to that extent. Even a partial loss of overweight is highly beneficial, and it is our experience that once a patient has completed a first course he is so enthusiastic about the ease with which the – to him surprising – results are achieved that he almost invariably comes back for more. There certainly can be no doubt that in my clinic more time is spent on damping over-enthusiasm than on insisting that the rules of the treatment be observed.

Examining the Patient

Only when agreement is reached on the points so far discussed do we proceed with the examination of the patient. A note is made of the size of the first upper incisor, of a pad of fat on the nape of the neck, at the axilla and on the inside of the knees. The presence of striation, a suprapubic fold, a thoracic fold, angulation of elbow and knee joint, breast-development in men and women, edema of the ankles and the state of genital development in the male are noted.

Wherever this seems indicated we X-ray the sella turcica, as the bony capsule which contains the pituitary gland is called, measure the basal metabolic rate, X-ray the chest and take an electrocardiogram. We do a blood-count and a sedimentation rate and estimate uric acid, cholesterol, iodine and sugar in the fasting blood.

Gain Before Loss

Patients whose general condition is low, owing to excessive previous dieting, must eat to capacity for about one week before starting treatment, regardless of how much weight they may gain in the process. One cannot keep a patient comfortably on 500 Calories unless his normal fat reserves are reasonably well stocked. **It is for**

this reason also that every case, even those that are actually gaining must eat to capacity of the most fattening food they can get down until they have had the third injection. It is a fundamental mistake to put a patient on 500 Calories as soon as the injections are started, as it seems to take about three injections before abnormally deposited fat begins to circulate and thus become available.

We distinguish between the first three injections, which we call "non-effective" as far as the loss of weight is concerned, and the subsequent injections given while the patient is dieting, which we call "effective". The average loss of weight is calculated on the number of effective injections and from the weight reached on the day of the third injection which may be well above what it was two days earlier when the first injection was given.

Most patients who have been struggling with diets for years and know how rapidly they gain if they let themselves go are very hard to convince of the absolute necessity of gorging for at least two days, and yet this must he insisted upon categorically if the further course of treatment is to run smoothly. Those patients who have to be put on forced feeding for a week before starting the injections usually gain weight rapidly – four to six pounds in 24 hours is not unusual – but after a day or two this rapid gain generally levels off. In any case, the whole gain is usually lost in the first 48 hours of dieting. It is necessary to proceed in this manner because the gain re-stocks the depleted normal reserves, whereas the subsequent loss is from the abnormal deposits only.

Patients in a satisfactory general condition and those who have not just previously restricted their diet start forced feeding on the day of the first injection. Some patents say that they can no longer overeat because their stomach has shrunk after years of restrictions. While we know that no stomach ever shrinks, we compromise by insisting that they eat frequently of highly concentrated foods such as milk chocolate, pastries with whipped cream sugar, fried meats (particularly pork), eggs and bacon, mayonnaise, bread with thick butter and jam, etc. The time and trouble spent on pressing this point upon incredulous or reluctant patients is always amply rewarded afterwards by the complete absence of those difficulties which patients who have disregarded these instructions are liable to experience.

During the two days of forced feeding from the first to the third injection – many patients are surprised that contrary to their previous experience they do not gain weight and some even lose. The explanation is that in these cases there is a compensatory flow of urine, which drains excessive water from the body. To some extent this seems to be a direct action of HCG, but it may also be due to a higher protein intake, as we know that a protein-deficient diet makes the body retain water.

Starting Treatment

In menstruating women, the best time to start treatment is immediately after a period. Treatment may also be started later, but it is advisable to have at least ten days in hand before the onset of the next period. Similarly, the end of a course of HCG should never be made to coincide with menstruation. If things should happen to work out that way, it is better to give the last injection three days before the expected date of the menses so that a normal diet can be resumed at onset. Alternatively, at least three injections should be given after the period, followed by the usual three days of dieting. This rule need not be observed in such patients who have reached their normal weight before the end of treatment and are already on a higher caloric diet.

Patients who require more than the minimum of 23 injections and who therefore skip one day a week in order to postpone immunity to HCG cannot have their third injections on the day before the interval. Thus if it is decided to skip Sundays, the treatment can be started on any day of the week except Thursdays. Supposing they start on Thursday, they will have their third injection on Saturday, which is also the day on which they start their 500 Calorie diet. They would then have no injection on the second day of dieting; this exposes them to an unnecessary hardship, as without the injection they will feel particularly hungry. Of course, the difficulty can be overcome by exceptionally injecting them on the first Sunday. If this day falls between the first and second or between the second and third injection, we usually prefer to give the patient the extra day of forced feeding, which the majority rapturously enjoy.

The Diet

The 500 Calorie diet is explained on the day of the second injection to those patients who will be preparing their own food, and it is most important that the person who will actually cook is present – the wife, the mother or the cook, as the case may be. Here in Italy patients are given the following diet sheet.

BREAKFAST: Tea or coffee in any quantity without sugar. Only one tablespoonful of milk allowed in 24 hours. Saccharin or other sweeteners may be used.

LUNCH:

1) 100 grams of veal, beef, chicken breast, fresh white fish, lobster, crab, or shrimp. All visible fat must be carefully removed before cooking, and the meat must be weighed raw. It must be boiled or grilled without additional fat. Salmon, eel, tuna, herring, dried or pickled fish are not allowed. The chicken breast must be removed raw from the bird.

2) One type of vegetable only to be chosen from the following: spinach, chard, chicory, beet-greens, green salad, tomatoes, celery, fennel, onions, red radishes, cucumbers, asparagus, cabbage.

3) One breadstick (grissino) or one Melba toast.

4) An apple or an orange or a handful of strawberries or one-half grapefruit.

DINNER: The same four choices as lunch.

The juice of one lemon daily is allowed for all purposes. Salt, pepper, vinegar, mustard powder, garlic, sweet basil, parsley, thyme, marjoram, etc., may be used for seasoning, but no oil, butter or dressing.

Tea, coffee, plain water, or mineral water are the only drinks allowed, but they may be taken in any quantity and at all times.

In fact, the patient should drink about 2 liters of these fluids per day. Many patients are afraid to drink so much because they fear that this may make them retain more water. This is a wrong notion as the body is more inclined to store water when the intake falls below its normal requirements.

The fruit or the breadstick may be eaten between meals instead of with lunch or dinner, but not more than four items listed for lunch and dinner may be eaten at one meal.

No medicines or cosmetics other than lipstick, eyebrow pencil and powder may be used without special permission.

Every item in the list is gone over carefully, continually stressing the point that no variations other than those listed may be introduced. All things not listed are forbidden, and the patient is assured that nothing permissible has been left out. The 100 grams of meat must he scrupulously weighed raw after all visible fat has been removed. To do this accurately the patient must have a letter-scale, as kitchen scales are not sufficiently accurate and the butcher should certainly not be relied upon. Those not uncommon patients who feel that even so little food is too much for them, can omit anything they wish.

There is no objection to breaking up the two meals. For instance having a breadstick and an apple for breakfast or an orange before going to bed, provided they are deducted from the regular meals. The whole daily ration of two breadsticks or two fruits may not be eaten at the same time, nor can any item saved from the previous day be added on the following day. In the beginning patients are advised to check every meal against their diet sheet before starting to eat and not to rely on their memory. It is also worth pointing out that any attempt to observe this diet without HCG will lead to trouble in two to three days. We have had cases in which patients have proudly flaunted their dieting powers in front of their friends without mentioning the fact that they are also receiving treatment with HCG. They let their friends try the same diet, and when this proves to be a failure – as it necessarily must – the patient starts raking in unmerited kudos for superhuman willpower.

It should also be mentioned that two small apples weighing as much as one large one never the less have a higher caloric value and are therefore not allowed though there is no restriction on the size of one apple. Some people do not realize that a tangerine is not an orange and that chicken breast does not mean the breast of any other fowl, nor does it mean a wing or drumstick.

The most tiresome patients are those who start counting Calories and then come up with all manner of ingenious variations which they compile from their little books. When one has spent years of weary research trying to make a diet as attractive as possible without jeopardizing the loss of weight, culinary geniuses who are out to improve their unhappy lot are hard to take.

Making Up the Calories

The diet used in conjunction with HCG must not exceed 500 Calories per day, and the way these Calories are made up is of utmost importance. For instance, if a patient drops the apple and eats an extra breadstick instead, he will not be getting more Calories but he will not lose weight. There are a number of foods, particularly fruits and vegetables, which have the same or even lower caloric values than those listed as permissible, and yet we find that they interfere with the regular loss of weight under HCG, presumably owing to the nature of their composition. Pimiento peppers, okra, artichokes and pears are examples of this.

While this diet works satisfactorily in Italy, certain modifications have to be made in other countries. For instance, American beef has almost double the caloric value of South Italian beef, which is not marbled with fat. This marbling is impossible to remove. In America, therefore, low-grade veal should be used for one meal and fish (excluding all those species such as herring, mackerel, tuna, salmon, eel, etc., which have a high fat content, and all dried, smoked or pickled fish), chicken breast, lobster, crawfish, prawns, shrimps, crabmeat or kidneys for the other meal. Where the Italian breadsticks, the so-called grissini, are not available, one Melba toast may be used instead, though they are psychologically less satisfying. A Melba toast has about the same weight as the very porous grissini which is much more to look at and to chew.

In many countries specially prepared unsweetened and low Calorie foods are freely available, and some of these can be tentatively used. When local conditions or the feeding habits of the population make changes necessary it must be borne in mind that the total daily intake must not exceed 500 Calories if the best possible results are to be obtained, that the daily ration should contain 200 grams of fat-free protein and a very small amount of starch.

Just as the daily dose of HCG is the same in all cases, so the same diet proves to be satisfactory for a small elderly lady of leisure or a hard working muscular giant. Under the effect of HCG the obese body is always able to obtain all the Calories it needs from the abnormal fat deposits, regardless of whether it uses up 1500 or 4000 per day. It must be made very clear to the patient that he is living to a far greater extent on the fat which he is losing than on what he eats.

Many patients ask why eggs are not allowed. The contents of two good sized eggs are roughly equivalent to 100 grams of meat, but unfortunately the yolk contains a large amount of fat, which is undesirable. Very occasionally we allow egg – boiled, poached or raw – to patients who develop an aversion to meat, but in this case they must add the white of three eggs to the one they eat whole. In countries where cottage cheese made from skimmed milk is available 100 grams may occasionally be used instead of the meat, but no other cheeses are allowed.

Vegetarians

Strict vegetarians such as orthodox Hindus present a special problem, because milk and curds are the only animal protein they will

52

eat. To supply them with sufficient protein of animal origin they must drink 500 cc. of skimmed milk per day, though part of this ration can be taken as curds. As far as fruit, vegetables and starch are concerned, their diet is the same as that of non-vegetarians; they cannot be allowed their usual intake of vegetable proteins from leguminous plants such as beans or from wheat or nuts, nor can they have their customary rice. In spite of these severe restrictions, their average loss is about half that of non-vegetarians, presumably owing to the sugar content of the milk.

Faulty Dieting

Few patients will take one's word for it that the slightest deviation from the diet has under HCG disastrous results as far as the weight is concerned. This extreme sensitivity has the advantage that the smallest error is immediately detectable at the daily weighing but most patients have to make the experience before they will believe it.

Persons in high official positions such as embassy personnel, politicians, senior executives, etc., who are obliged to attend social functions to which they cannot bring their meager meal must be told beforehand that an official dinner will cost them the loss of about three days treatment, however careful they are and in spite of a friendly and would-be cooperative host. We generally advise them to avoid all-round embarrassment, the almost inevitable turn of conversation to their weight problem and the outpouring of lay counsel from their table partners by not letting it be known that they are under treatment. They should take dainty servings of everything, hide what they can under the cutlery and book the gain which may take three days to get rid of as one of the sacrifices which their profession entails. Allowing three days for their correction, such incidents do not jeopardize the treatment, provided they do not occur all too frequently in which case treatment should be postponed to a socially more peaceful season.

Vitamins and Anemia

Sooner or later most patients express a fear that they may be running out of vitamins or that the restricted diet may make them anemic. On this score the physician can confidently relieve their apprehension by explaining that every time they lose a pound of fatty tissue, which they do almost daily, only the actual fat is burned up; all the vitamins, the proteins, the blood, and the minerals which this tissue contains in abundance are fed back into the body. Actually, a low blood count not due to any serious disorder of the blood forming

53

tissues improves during treatment, and we have never encountered a significant protein deficiency nor signs of a lack of vitamins in patients who are dieting regularly.

The First Days of Treatment

On the day of the third injection it is almost routine to hear two remarks. One is: "You know, Doctor, I'm sure it's only psychological, but I already feel quite different." So common is this remark, even from very skeptical patients that we hesitate to accept the psychological interpretation. The other typical remark is: "Now that I have been allowed to eat anything I want, I can't get it down. Since yesterday I feel like a stuffed pig. Food just doesn't seem to interest me any more, and I am longing to get on with your diet." Many patients notice that they are passing more urine and that the swelling in their ankles is less even before they start dieting.

On the day of the fourth injection most patients declare that they are feeling fine. They have usually lost two pounds or more, some say they feel a bit empty but hasten to explain that this does not amount to hunger. Some complain of a mild headache of which they have been forewarned and for which they have been given permission to take aspirin.

During the second and third day of dieting – that is, the fifth and sixth injection – these minor complaints improve while the weight continues to drop at about double the usually overall average of almost one pound per day, so that a moderately severe case may by the fourth day of dieting have lost as much as 8-10 lbs.

It is usually at this point that a difference appears between those patients who have literally eaten to capacity during the first two days of treatment and those who have not. The former feel remarkably well; they have no hunger, nor do they feel tempted when others eat normally at the same table. They feel lighter, more clear-headed and notice a desire to move quite contrary to their previous lethargy. Those who have disregarded the advice to eat to capacity continue to have minor discomforts and do not have the same euphoric sense of well-being until about a week later. It seems that their normal fat reserves require that much more time before they are fully stocked.

Fluctuations in Weight Loss

After the fourth or fifth day of dieting the daily loss of weight begins to decrease to one pound or somewhat less per day, and there is a smaller urinary output. Men often continue to lose regularly at

54

that rate, but women are more irregular in spite of faultless dieting. There may be no drop at all for two or three days and then a sudden loss which reestablishes the normal average. These fluctuations are entirely due to variations in the retention and elimination of water, which are more marked in women than in men.

The weight registered by the scale is determined by two processes not necessarily synchronized. Under the influence of HCG, fat is being extracted from the cells, in which it is stored in the fatty tissue. When these cells are empty and therefore serve no purpose, the body breaks down the cellular structure and absorbs it, but breaking up of useless cells, connective tissue, blood vessels, etc., may lag behind the process of fat-extraction. When this happens the body appears to replace some of the extracted fat with water which is retained for this purpose. As water is heavier than fat the scales may show no loss of weight, although sufficient fat has actually been consumed to make up for the deficit in the 500-Calorie diet. When then such tissue is finally broken down, the water is liberated and there is a sudden flood of urine and a marked loss of weight. This simple interpretation of what is really an extremely complex mechanism is the one we give those patients who want to know why it is that on certain days they do not lose, though they have committed no dietary error.

Patients who have previously regularly used diuretics as a method of reducing, lose fat during the first two or three weeks of treatment which shows in their measurements, but the scale may show little or no loss because they are replacing the normal water content of their body which has been dehydrated. Diuretics should never be used for reducing.

Interruptions of Weight Loss

We distinguish four types of interruption in the regular daily loss. The first is the one that has already been mentioned in which the weight stays stationary for a day or two, and this occurs, particularly towards the end of a course, in almost every case.

The Plateau

The second type of interruption we call a "plateau." A plateau lasts 4-6 days and frequently occurs during the second half of a full course, particularly in patients that have been doing well and whose overall average of nearly a pound per effective injection has been maintained. Those who are losing more than the average all have a plateau sooner or later. A plateau always corrects, itself, but many patients who have become accustomed to a regular daily loss get unnecessarily worried and begin to fret. No amount of explanation convinces them that a plateau does not mean that they are no longer responding normally to treatment.

In such cases we consider it permissible, for purely psychological reasons, to break up the plateau. This can be done in two ways. One is a so-called "apple day." An apple-day begins at lunch and continues until just before lunch of the following day. The patients are given six large apples and are told to eat one whenever they feel the desire though six apples is the maximum allowed. During an apple-day no other food or liquids except plain water are allowed and of water they may only drink just enough to quench an uncomfortable thirst if eating an apple still leaves them thirsty. Most patients feel no need for water and are quite happy with their six apples. Needless to say, an apple-day may never be given on the day on which there is no injection. The apple-day produces a gratifying loss of weight on the following day, chiefly due to the elimination of water. This water is not regained when the patients resume their normal 500-Calorie diet at lunch, and on the following days they continue to lose weight satisfactorily.

The other way to break up a plateau is by giving a non-mercurial diuretic[7] for one day. This is simpler for the patient but we prefer the apple-day as we sometimes find that though the diuretic is very effective on the following day it may take two to three days before the normal daily reduction is resumed, throwing the patient into a new fit of despair. It is useless to give either an apple-day or a diuretic unless the weight has been stationary for at least four days without any dietary error having been committed.

Reaching a Former Level

The third type of interruption in the regular loss of weight may last much longer — ten days to two weeks. Fortunately, it is rare and only occurs in very advanced cases, and then hardly ever during the first course of treatment. It is seen only in those patients who during some period of their lives have maintained a certain fixed degree of obesity for ten years or more and have then at some time rapidly increased beyond that weight. When then in the course of treatment the former level is reached, it may take two weeks of no

---

[7] We use 1 tablet of hygroton.

loss, in spite of HCG and diet, before further reduction is normally resumed.

Menstrual Interruption

The fourth type of interruption is the one which often occurs a few days before and during the menstrual period and in some women at the time of ovulation. It must also be mentioned that when a woman becomes pregnant during treatment – and this is by no means uncommon – she at once ceases to lose weight. An unexplained arrest of reduction has on several occasions raised our suspicion before the first period was missed. If in such cases, menstruation is delayed, we stop injecting and do a precipitation test five days later. No pregnancy test should be carried out earlier than five days after the last injection, as otherwise the HCG may give a false positive result.

Oral contraceptives may be used during treatment.

Dietary Errors

Any interruption of the normal loss of weight which does not fit perfectly into one of those categories is always due to some possibly very minor dietary error. Similarly, any gain of more than 100 grams is invariably the result of some transgression or mistake, unless it happens on or about the day of ovulation or during the three days preceding the onset of menstruation, in which case it is ignored. In all other cases the reason for the gain must be established at once.

The patient who frankly admits that he has stepped out of his regimen when told that something has gone wrong is no problem. He is always surprised at being found out, because unless he has seen this himself he will not believe that a salted almond, a couple of potato chips, a glass of tomato juice or an extra orange will bring about a definite increase in his weight on the following day.

Very often he wants to know why extra food weighing one ounce should increase his weight by six ounces. We explain this in the following way: Under the influence of HCG the blood is saturated with food and the blood volume has adapted itself so that it can only just accommodate the 500 Calories which come in from the intestinal tract in the course of the day. Any additional income, however little this may be, cannot be accommodated and the blood is therefore forced to increase its volume sufficiently to hold the extra food, which it can only do in a very diluted form. Thus it is not the weight of what is eaten that plays the determining role but rather the amount of water which the body must retain to accommodate this food.

This can be illustrated by mentioning the case of salt. In order to hold one teaspoonful of salt the body requires one liter of water, as it cannot accommodate salt in any higher concentration. Thus, if a person eats one teaspoonful of salt his weight will go up by more than two pounds as soon as this salt is absorbed from his intestine.

To this explanation many patients reply: Well, if I put on that much every time I eat a little extra, how can I hold my weight after the treatment? It must therefore be made clear that this only happens as long as they are under HCG. When treatment is over, the blood is no longer saturated and can easily accommodate extra food without having to increase its volume. Here again the professional reader will be aware that this interpretation is a simplification of an extremely intricate physiological process which actually accounts for the phenomenon.

Salt and Reducing

While we are on the subject of salt, I can take this opportunity to explain that we make no restriction in the use of salt and insist that the patients drink large quantities of water throughout the treatment. We are out to reduce abnormal fat and are not in the least interested in such illusory weight losses as can be achieved by depriving the body of salt and by desiccating it. Though we allow the free use of salt, the daily amount taken should be roughly the same, as a sudden increase will of course be followed by a corresponding increase in weight as shown by the scale. An increase in the intake of salt is one of the most common causes for an increase in weight from one day to the next. Such an increase can be ignored, provided it is accounted for. It in no way influences the regular loss of fat.

Water

Patients are usually hard to convince that the amount of water they retain has nothing to do with the amount of water they drink. When the body is forced to retain water, it will do this at all costs. If the fluid intake is insufficient to provide all the water required, the body withholds water from the kidneys and the urine becomes scanty and highly concentrated, imposing a certain strain on the kidneys. If that is insufficient, excessive water will be with-drawn from the intestinal tract, with the result that the feces become hard and dry. On the other hand if a patient drinks more than his body requires, the surplus is promptly and easily eliminated. Trying to prevent the body from retaining water by drinking less is therefore not only futile but even harmful.

58

Constipation

An excess of water keeps the feces soft, and that is very important in the obese, who commonly suffer from constipation and a spastic colon. While a patient is under treatment we never permit the use of any kind of laxative taken by mouth. We explain that owing to the restricted diet it is perfectly satisfactory and normal to have an evacuation of the bowel only once every three to four days and that, provided plenty of fluids are taken, this never leads to any disturbance. Only in those patients who begin to fret after four days do we allow the use of a suppository. Patients who observe this rule find that after treatment they have a perfectly normal bowel action and this delights many of them almost as much as their loss of weight.

Investigating Dietary Errors

When the reason for a slight gain in weight is not immediately evident, it is necessary to investigate further. A patient who is unaware of having committed an error or is unwilling to admit a mistake protests indignantly when told he has done something he ought not to have done. In that atmosphere no fruitful investigation can be conducted; so we calmly explain that we are not accusing him of anything but that we know for certain from our not inconsiderable experience that something has gone wrong and that we must now sit down quietly together and try and find out what it was. Once the patient realizes that it is in his own interest that he play an active and not merely a passive role in this search, the reason for the setback is almost invariably discovered. Having been through hundreds of such sessions, we are nearly always able to distinguish the deliberate liar from the patient who is merely fooling himself or is really unaware of having erred.

Liars and Fools

When we see obese patients there are generally two of us present in order to speed up routine handling. Thus when we have to investigate a rise in weight, a glance is sufficient to make sure that we agree or disagree. If after a few questions we both feel reasonably sure that the patient is deliberately lying, we tell him that this is our opinion and warn him that unless he comes clean we may refuse further treatment. The way he reacts to this furnishes additional proof whether we are on the right track or not; we now very rarely make a mistake.

If the patient breaks down and confesses, we melt and are all forgiveness and treatment proceeds. Yet if such performances have to be repeated more than two or three times, we refuse further treatment. This happens in less than 1% of our cases. If the patient is stubborn and will not admit what he has been up to, we usually give him one more chance and continue treatment even though we have been unable to find the reason for his gain. In many such cases there is no repetition, and frequently the patient does then confess a few days later after he has thought things over.

The patient who is fooling himself is the one who has committed some trifling, offense against the rules but who has been able to convince himself that this is of no importance and cannot possibly account for the gain in weight. Women seem particularly prone to getting themselves entangled in such delusions. On the other hand, it does frequently happen that a patient will in the midst of a conversation unthinkingly spear an olive or forget that he has already eaten his breadstick.

A mother preparing food for the family may out of sheer habit forget that she must not taste the sauce to see whether it needs more salt. Sometimes a rich maiden aunt cannot be offended by refusing a cup of tea into which she has put two teaspoons of sugar, thoughtfully remembering the patient's taste from previous occasions. Such incidents are legion and are usually confessed without hesitation, but some patients seem genuinely able to forget these lapses and remember them with a visible shock only after insistent questioning.

In these cases we go carefully over the day. Sometimes the patient has been invited to a meal or gone to a restaurant, naively believing that the food has actually been prepared exactly according to instructions. They will say: "Yes, now that I come to think of it the steak did seem a bit bigger than the one I have at home, and it did taste better; maybe there was a little fat on it, though I specially told them to cut it all away." Sometimes the breadsticks were broken and a few fragments eaten, and "Maybe they were a little more than one." It is not uncommon for patients to place too much reliance on their memory of the diet-sheet and start eating carrots, beans or peas and then to seem genuinely surprised when their attention is called to the fact that these are forbidden, as they have not been listed.

Cosmetics

When no dietary error is elicited we turn to cosmetics. Most women find it hard to believe that fats, oils, creams and ointments

60

applied to the skin are absorbed and interfere with weight reduction by HCG just as if they had been eaten. This almost incredible sensitivity to even such very minor increases in nutritional intake is a peculiar feature of the HCG method. For instance, we find that persons who habitually handle organic fats, such as workers in beauty parlors, masseurs, butchers, etc. never show what we consider a satisfactory loss of weight unless they can avoid fat coming into contact with their skin.

The point is so important that I will illustrate it with two cases. A lady who was cooperating perfectly suddenly increased half a pound. Careful questioning brought nothing to light. She had certainly made no dietary error nor had she used any kind of face cream, and she was already in the menopause. As we felt that we could trust her implicitly, we left the question suspended. Yet just as she was about to leave the consulting room she suddenly stopped, turned and snapped her fingers. "I've got it," she said. This is what had happened : She had bought herself a new set of make-up pots and bottles and, using her fingers, had transferred her large assortment of cosmetics to the new containers in anticipation of the day she would be able to use them again after her treatment.

The other case concerns a man who impressed us as being very conscientious. He was about 20 lbs. overweight but did not lose satisfactorily from the onset of treatment. Again and again we tried to find the reason but with no success, until one day he said: "I never told you this, but I have a glass eye. In fact, I have a whole set of them. I frequently change them, and every time I do that I put a special ointment in my eyesocket. Do you think that could have anything to do with it?" As we thought just that, we asked him to stop using this ointment, and from that day on his weight-loss was regular.

We are particularly averse to those modern cosmetics which contain hormones, as any interference with endocrine regulations during treatment must be absolutely avoided. Many women whose skin has in the course of years become adjusted to the use of fat containing cosmetics find that their skin gets dry as soon as they stop using them. In such cases we permit the use of plain mineral oil, which has no nutritional value. On the other hand, mineral oil should not be used in preparing the food, first because of its undesirable laxative quality, and second because it absorbs some fat-soluble vitamins, which are then lost in the stool. We do permit the use of lipstick, powder and such lotions as are entirely free of fatty substances. We also allow brilliantine to be used on the hair but it must not be rubbed into the scalp. Obviously sun-tan oil is prohibited.

Many women are horrified when told that for the duration of treatment they cannot use face creams or have facial massages. They fear that this and the loss of weight will ruin their complexion. They can be fully reassured. Under treatment normal fat is restored to the skin, which rapidly becomes fresh and turgid, making the expression much more youthful. This is a characteristic of the HCG method which is a constant source of wonder to patients who have experienced or seen in others the facial ravages produced by the usual methods of reducing. An obese woman of 70 obviously cannot expect to have her pued face reduced to normal without a wrinkle, but it is remarkable how youthful her face remains in spite of her age.

The Voice

Incidentally, another interesting feature of the HCG method is that it does not ruin a singing voice. The typically obese prima donna usually finds that when she tries to reduce, the timbre of her voice is liable to change, and understandably this terrifies her. Under HCG this does not happen; indeed, in many cases the voice improves and the breathing invariably does. We have had many cases of professional singers very carefully controlled by expert voice teachers, and the maestros have been so enthusiastic that they now frequently send us patients.

Other Reasons for a Gain

Apart from diet and cosmetics there can be a few other reasons for a small rise in weight. Some patients unwittingly take chewing gum, throat pastilles, vitamin pills, cough syrups etc., without realizing that the sugar or fats they contain may interfere with a regular loss of weight. Sex hormones or cortisone in its various modern forms must be avoided, though oral contraceptives are permitted. In fact the only self-medication we allow is aspirin for a headache, though headaches almost invariably disappear after a week of treatment, particularly if of the migraine type.

Occasionally we allow a sleeping tablet or a tranquilizer, but patients should be told that while under treatment they need and may get less sleep. For instance, here in Italy where it is customary to sleep during the siesta which lasts from one to four in the afternoon most patients find that though they lie down they are unable to sleep.

We encourage swimming and sun bathing during treatment, but it should be remembered that a severe sunburn always produces a temporary rise in weight, evidently due to water retention. The same may be seen when a patient gets a common cold during treatment.

62

Finally, the weight can temporarily increase – paradoxical though this may sound – after an exceptional physical exertion of long duration leading to a feeling of exhaustion. A game of tennis, a vigorous swim, a run, a ride on horseback or a round of golf do not have this effect; but a long trek, a day of skiing, rowing or cycling or dancing into the small hours usually result in a gain of weight on the following day, unless the patient is in perfect training. In patients coming from abroad, where they always use their cars, we often see this effect after a strenuous day of shopping on foot, sightseeing and visits to galleries and museums. Though the extra muscular effort involved does consume some additional Calories, this appears to be offset by the retention of water which the tired circulation cannot at once eliminate.

Appetite-reducing Drugs

We hardly ever use amphetamines, the appetite-reducing drugs such as Dexedrin, Dexamil, Preludin, etc., as there seems to be no need for them during the HCG treatment. The only time we find them useful is when a patient is, for impelling and unforeseen reasons, obliged to forego the injections for three to four days and yet wishes to continue the diet so that he need not interrupt the course.

Unforeseen Interruptions of Treatment

If an interruption of treatment lasting more than four days is necessary, the patient must increase his diet to at least 800 Calories by adding meat, eggs, cheese, and milk to his diet after the third day, as otherwise he will find himself so hungry and weak that he is unable to go about his usual occupation. If the interval lasts less than two weeks the patient can directly resume injections and the 500-Calorie diet, but if the interruption lasts longer he must again eat normally until he has had his third injection.

When a patient knows beforehand that he will have to travel and be absent for more than four days, it is always better to stop injections three days before he is due to leave so that he can have the three days of strict dieting which are necessary after the last injection at home. This saves him from the almost impossible task of having to arrange the 500 Calorie diet while en route, and he can thus enjoy a much greater dietary freedom from the day of his departure. Interruptions occurring before 20 effective injections have been given are most undesirable, because with less than that number of injections some weight is liable to be regained. After the 20th injection an unavoidable interruption is merely a loss of time.

Muscular Fatigue

Towards the end of a full course, when a good deal of fat has been rapidly lost, some patients complain that lifting a weight or climbing stairs requires a greater muscular effort than before. They feel neither breathlessness nor exhaustion but simply that their muscles have to work harder. This phenomenon, which disappears soon after the end of the treatment, is caused by the removal of abnormal fat deposited between, in, and around the muscles. The removal of this fat makes the muscles too long, and so in order to achieve a certain skeletal movement – say the bending of an arm – the muscles have to perform greater contraction than before. Within a short while the muscle adjusts itself perfectly to the new situation, but under HCG the loss of fat is so rapid that this adjustment cannot keep up with it. Patients often have to be reassured that this does not mean that they are "getting weak." This phenomenon does not occur in patients who regularly take vigorous exercise and continue to do so during treatment.

Massage

I never allow any kind of massage during treatment. It is entirely unnecessary and merely disturbs a very delicate process which is going on in the tissues. Few indeed are the masseurs and masseuses who can resist the temptation to knead and hammer abnormal fat deposits. In the course of rapid reduction it is sometimes possible to pick up a fold of skin which has not yet had time to adjust itself, as it always does under HCG, to the changed figure. This fold contains its normal subcutaneous fat and may be almost an inch thick. It is one of the main objects of the HCG treatment to keep that fat there. Patients and their masseurs do not always understand this and give this fat a working-over. I have seen such patients who were as black and blue as if they had received a sound thrashing.

In my opinion, massage, thumping, rolling, kneading, and shivering undertaken for the purpose of reducing abnormal fat can do nothing but harm. We once had the honor of treating the proprietress of a high class institution that specialized in such antics. She had the audacity to confess that she was taking our treatment to convince her clients of the efficacy of her methods, which she had found useless in her own case.

How anyone in his right mind is able to believe that fatty tissue can be shifted mechanically or be made to vanish by squeezing is beyond my comprehension. The only effect obtained is severe

64

bruising. The torn tissue then forms scars, and these slowly contract making the fatty tissue even harder and more unyielding.

A lady once consulted us for her most ungainly legs. Large masses of fat bulged over the ankles of her tiny feet, and there were about 40 lbs. too much on her hips and thighs. We assured her that this overweight could be lost and that her ankles would markedly improve in the process. Her treatment progressed most satisfactorily but to our surprise there was no improvement in her ankles. We then discovered that she had for years been taking every kind of mechanical, electric and heat treatment for her legs and that she had made up her mind to resort to plastic surgery if we failed.

Re-examining the fat above her ankles, we found that it was unusually hard. We attributed this to the countless minor injuries inflicted by kneading. These injuries had healed but had left a tough network of connective scar-tissue in which the fat was imprisoned. Ready to try anything, she was put to bed for the remaining three weeks of her first course with her lower legs tightly strapped in unyielding bandages. Every day the pressure was increased. The combination of HCG, diet and strapping brought about a marked improvement in the shape of her ankles. At the end of her first course she returned to her home abroad. Three months later she came back for her second course. She had maintained both her weight and the improvement of her ankles. The same procedure was repeated, and after five weeks she left the hospital with a normal weight and legs that, if not exactly shapely, were at least unobtrusive. Where no such injuries of the tissues have been inflicted by inappropriate methods of treatment, these drastic measures are never necessary.

Blood Sugar

Towards the end of a course or when a patient has nearly reached his normal weight it occasionally happens that the blood sugar drops below normal, and we have even seen this in patients who had an abnormally high blood sugar before treatment. Such an attack of hypoglycemia is almost identical with the one seen in diabetics who have taken too much insulin. The attack comes on suddenly; there is the same feeling of light-headedness, weakness in the knees, trembling, and unmotivated sweating; but under HCG, hypoglycemia does not produce any feeling of hunger. All these symptoms are almost instantly relieved by taking two heaped teaspoons of sugar.

In the course of treatment the possibility of such an attack is explained to those patients who are in a phase in which a drop in blood sugar may occur. They are instructed to keep sugar or glucose sweets handy, particularly when driving a car. They are also told to watch the effect of taking sugar very carefully and report the following day. This is important, because anxious patients to whom such an attack has been explained are apt to take sugar unnecessarily, in which case it inevitably produces a gain in weight and does not dramatically relieve the symptoms for which it was taken, proving that these were not due to hypoglycemia. Some patients mistake the effects of emotional stress for hypoglycemia. When the symptoms are quickly relieved by sugar this is proof that they were indeed due to an abnormal lowering of the blood sugar, and in that case there is no increase in the weight on the following day. We always suggest that sugar be taken if the patient is in doubt.

Once such an attack has been relieved with sugar we have never seen it recur on the immediately subsequent days, and only very rarely does a patient have two such attacks separated by several days during a course of treatment. In patients who have not eaten sufficiently during the first two days of treatment we sometimes give sugar when the minor symptoms usually felt during the first three days of treatment continue beyond that time, and in some cases this has seemed to speed up the euphoria ordinarily associated with the HCG method.

The Ratio of Pounds to Inches

An interesting feature of the HCG method is that, regardless of how fat a patient is, the greatest circumference — abdomen or hips as the case may be is reduced at a constant rate which is extraordinarily close to 1 cm. per kilogram of weight lost. At the beginning of treatment the change in measurements is somewhat greater than this, but at the end of a course it is almost invariably found that the girth is as many centimeters less as the number of kilograms by which the weight has been reduced. I have never seen this clear cut relationship in patients that try to reduce by dieting only.

Preparing the Solution

Human chorionic gonadotrophin comes on the market as a highly soluble powder which is the pure substance extracted from the urine of pregnant women. Such preparations are carefully standardized, and any brand made by a reliable pharmaceutical company is probably as good as any other. The substance should be extracted from the urine and not from the placenta, and it must of

66

course be of human and not of animal origin. The powder is sealed in ampoules or in rubber-capped bottles in varying amounts which are stated in International Units. In this form HCG is stable; however, only such preparations should be used that have the date of manufacture and the date of expiry clearly stated on the label or package. A suitable solvent is always supplied in a separate ampoule in the same package.

Once HCG is in solution it is far less stable. It may be kept at room-temperature for two to three days, but if the solution must be kept longer it should always be refrigerated. When treating only one or two cases simultaneously, vials containing a small number of units say 1000 I.U. should be used. The 10 cc. of solvent which is supplied by the manufacturer is injected into the rubber- capped bottle containing the HCG, and the powder must dissolve instantly. Of this solution 1.25 cc. are withdrawn for each injection. One such bottle of 1000 I.U. therefore furnishes 8 injections. When more than one patient is being treated, they should not each have their own bottle but rather all be injected from the same vial and a fresh solution made when this is empty.

As we are usually treating a fair number of patients at the same time, we prefer to use vials containing 5000 units. With these the manufactures also supply 10 cc. of solvent. Of such a solution 0.25 cc. contain the 125 I.U., which is the standard dose for all cases and which should never be exceeded. This small amount is awkward to handle accurately (it requires an insulin syringe) and is wasteful, because there is a loss of solution in the nozzle of the syringe and in the needle. We therefore prefer a higher dilution, which we prepare in the following way: The solvent supplied is injected into the rubber-capped bottle containing the 5000 I.U. As these bottles are too small to hold more solvent, we withdraw 5 cc., inject it into an empty rubber-capped bottle and add 5 cc. of normal saline to each bottle. This gives us 10 cc. of solution in each bottle, and of this solution 0.5 cc. contains 125 I.U. This amount is convenient to inject with an ordinary syringe.

Injecting
HCG produces little or no tissue-reaction, it is completely painless and in the many thousands of injections we have given we have never seen an inflammatory or suppurative reaction at the site of the injection.

One should avoid leaving a vacuum in the bottle after preparing the solution or after withdrawal of the amount required for the injections as otherwise alcohol used for sterilizing a frequently perforated rubber cap might be drawn into the solution. When sharp needles are used, it sometimes happens that a little bit of rubber is punched out of the rubber cap and can be seen as a small black speck floating in the solution. As these bits of rubber are heavier than the solution they rapidly settle out, and it is thus easy to avoid drawing them into the syringe.

We use very fine needles that are two inches long and inject deep intragluteally in the outer upper quadrant of the buttocks. The injection should if possible not be given into the superficial fat layers, which in very obese patients must be compressed so as to enable the needle to reach the muscle. Obviously needles and syringes must be carefully washed, sterilized and handled aseptically.[8] It is also important that the daily injection should be given at intervals as close to 24 hours as possible. Any attempt to economize in time by giving larger doses at longer intervals is doomed to produce less satisfactory results.

There are hardly any contraindications to the HCG method. Treatment can be continued in the presence of abscesses, suppuration, large infected wounds and major fractures. Surgery and general anesthesia are no reason to stop and we have given treatment during a severe attack of malaria. Acne or boils are no contraindication; the former usually clears up, and furunculosis comes to an end. Thrombophlebitis is no contraindication, and we have treated several obese patients with HCG and the 500-Calorie diet while suffering from this condition. Our impression has been that in obese patients the phlebitis does rather better and certainly no worse than under the usual treatment alone. This also applies to patients suffering from varicose ulcers which tend to heal rapidly.

Fibroids

While uterine fibroids seem to be in no way affected by HCG in the doses we use, we have found that very large, externally palpable uterine myomas are apt to give trouble. We are convinced that this is entirely due to the rather sudden disappearance of fat from the pelvic bed upon which they rest and that it is the weight of the tumor pressing on the underlying tissues which accounts for the

---

[8] NOTE: This practice is obsolete. Modern sanitary methods dictate throwing away used needles and syringes and using new ones for each injection.

discomfort or pain which may arise during treatment. While we disregard even fair-sized or multiple myomas, we insist that very large ones be operated before treatment. We have had patients present themselves for reducing fat from their abdomen who showed no signs of obesity, but had a large abdominal tumor.

Gallstones

Small stones in the gall bladder may in patients who have recently had typical colics cause more frequent colics under treatment with HCG. This may be due to the almost complete absence of fat from the diet, which prevents the normal emptying of the gall bladder. Before undertaking treatment we explain to such patients that there is a risk of more frequent and possibly severe symptoms and that it may become necessary to operate. If they are prepared to take this risk and provided they agree to undergo an operation if we consider this imperative, we proceed with treatment, as after weight reduction with HCG the operative risk is considerably reduced in an obese patient. In such cases we always give a drug which stimulates the flow of bile, and in the majority of cases nothing untoward happens. On the other hand, we have looked for and not found any evidence to suggest that the HCG treatment leads to the formation of gallstones as pregnancy sometimes does.

The Heart

Disorders of the heart are not as a rule contraindications. In fact, the removal of abnormal fat – particularly from the heart-muscle and from the surrounding of the coronary arteries – can only be beneficial in cases of myocardial weakness, and many such patients are referred to us by cardiologists. Within the first week of treatment all patients – not only heart cases – remark that they have lost much of their breathlessness

Coronary Occlusion

In obese patients who have recently survived a coronary occlusion, we adopt the following procedure in collaboration with the cardiologist. We wait until no further electrocardiographic changes have occurred for a period of three months. Routine treatment is then started under careful control and it is usual to find a further electrocardiographic improvement of a condition which was previously stationary.

In the thousands of cases we have treated we have not once seen any sort of coronary incident occur during or shortly after treatment. The same applies to cerebral vascular accidents. Nor have we ever seen a case of thrombosis of any sort develop during treatment, even though a high blood pressure is rapidly lowered. In this respect, too, the HCG treatment resembles pregnancy.

Teeth and Vitamins

Patients whose teeth are in poor repair sometimes get more trouble under prolonged treatment, just as may occur in pregnancy. In such cases we do allow calcium and vitamin D, though not in an oily solution. The only other vitamin we permit is vitamin C, which we use in large doses combined with an antihistamine at the onset of a common cold. There is no objection to the use of an antibiotic if this is required, for instance by the dentist. In cases of bronchial asthma and hay fever we have occasionally resorted to cortisone during treatment and find that triamcinolone is the least likely to interfere with the loss of weight, but many asthmatics improve with HCG alone.

Alcohol

Obese heavy drinkers, even those bordering on alcoholism, often do surprisingly well under HCG and it is exceptional for them to take a drink while under treatment. When they do, they find that a relatively small quantity of alcohol produces intoxication. Such patients say that they do not feel the need to drink. This may in part be due to the euphoria which the treatment produces and in part to the complete absence of the need for quick sustenance from which most obese patients suffer.

Though we have had a few cases that have continued abstinence long after treatment, others relapse as soon as they are back on a normal diet. We have a few "regular customers" who, having once been reduced to their normal weight, start to drink again though watching their weight. Then after some months they purposely overeat in order to gain sufficient weight for another course of HCG which temporarily gets them out of their drinking routine. We do not particularly welcome such cases, but we see no reason for refusing their request.

Tuberculosis

It is interesting that obese patients suffering from inactive pulmonary tuberculosis can be safely treated. We have under very careful control treated patients as early as three months after they were pronounced inactive and have never seen a relapse occur during

70

or shortly after treatment. In fact, we only have one case on our records in which active tuberculosis developed in a young man about one year after a treatment which had lasted three weeks. Earlier X-rays showed a calcified spot from a childhood infection which had not produced clinical symptoms. There was a family history of tuberculosis, and his illness started under adverse conditions which certainly had nothing to do with the treatment. Residual calcifications from an early infection are exceedingly common, and we never consider them a contraindication to treatment.

The Painful Heel

In obese patients who have been trying desperately to keep their weight down by severe dieting, a curious symptom sometimes occurs. They complain of an unbearable pain in their heels which they feel only while standing or walking. As soon as they take the weight off their heels the pain ceases. These cases are the bane of the rheumatologists and orthopedic surgeons who have treated them before they come to us. All the usual investigations are entirely negative, and there is not the slightest response to anti- rheumatic medication or physiotherapy. The pain may be so severe that the patients are obliged to give up their occupation, and they are not infrequently labeled as a case of hysteria. When their heels are carefully examined one finds that the sole is softer than normal and that the heel bone – the calcaneus – can be distinctly felt, which is not the case in a normal foot.

We interpret the condition as a lack of the hard fatty pad on which the calcaneus rests and which protects both the bone and the skin of the sole from pressure. This fat is like a springy cushion which carries the weight of the body. Standing on a heel in which this fat is missing or reduced must obviously be very painful. In their efforts to keep their weight down these patients have consumed this normal structural fat.

Those patients who have a normal or subnormal weight while showing the typically obese fat deposits are made to eat to capacity, often much against their will, for one week. They gain weight rapidly but there is no improvement in the painful heels. They are then started on the routine HCG treatment. Overweight patients are treated immediately. In both cases the pain completely disappears in 10-20 days of dieting, usually around the 15th day of treatment, and so far no case has had a relapse though we have been able to follow up such patients for years.

We are particularly interested in these cases, as they furnish further proof of the contention that HCG + 500 Calories not only removes abnormal fat but actually permits normal fat to be replaced, in spite of the deficient food intake. It is certainly not so that the mere loss of weight reduces the pain, because it frequently disappears before the weight the patient had prior to the period of forced feeding is reached.

The Skeptical Patient

Any doctor who starts using the HCG method for the first time will have considerable difficulty, particularly if he himself is not fully convinced, in making patients believe that they will not feel hungry on 500 Calories and that their face will not collapse. New patients always anticipate the phenomena they know so well from previous treatments and diets and are incredulous when told that these will not occur. We overcome all this by letting new patients spend a little time in the waiting room with older hands, who can always be relied upon to allay these fears with evangelistic zeal, often demonstrating the finer points on their own body.

A waiting-room filled with obese patients who congregate daily is a sort of group therapy. They compare notes and pop back into the waiting room after the consultation to announce the score of the last 24 hours to an enthralled audience. They cross-check on their diets and sometimes confess sins which they try to hide from us, usually with the result that the patient in whom they have confided palpitatingly tattles the whole disgraceful story to us with a "But don't let her know I told you."

Concluding a Course

When the three days of dieting after the last injection are over, the patients are told that they may now eat anything they please, except sugar and starch provided they faithfully observe one simple rule. This rule is that they must have their own portable bathroom-scale always at hand, particularly while traveling. They must without fail weigh themselves every morning as they get out of bed, having first emptied their bladder. If they are in the habit of having breakfast in bed, they must weigh before breakfast.

It takes about 3 weeks before the weight reached at the end of the treatment becomes stable, i.e. does not show violent fluctuations after an occasional excess. During this period patients must realize that the so-called carbohydrates, that is sugar, rice, bread, potatoes, pastries, etc, are by far the most dangerous. If no carbohydrates

72

whatsoever are eaten, fats can be indulged in somewhat more liberally and even small quantities of alcohol, such as a glass of wine with meals, does no harm, but **as soon as fats and starch are combined things are very liable to get out of hand.** This has to be observed very carefully during the first 3 weeks after the treatment is ended otherwise disappointments are almost sure to occur.

Skipping a Meal

As long as their weight stays within two pounds of the weight reached on the day of the last injection, patients should take no notice of any increase but the moment the scale goes beyond two pounds, even if this is only a few ounces, they must on that same day entirely skip breakfast and lunch but take plenty to drink. In the evening they must eat a huge steak with only an apple or a raw tomato. Of course this rule applies only to the morning weight. Ex-obese patients should never check their weight during the day, as there may be wide fluctuations and these are merely alarming and confusing.

It is of utmost importance that the meal is skipped on the same day as the scale registers an increase of more than two pounds and that missing the meals is not postponed until the following day. If a meal is skipped on the day in which a gain is registered in the morning this brings about an immediate drop of often over a pound. But if the skipping of the meal – and skipping means literally skipping, not just having a light meal – is postponed the phenomenon does not occur and several days of strict dieting may be necessary to correct the situation.

Most patients hardly ever need to skip a meal. If they have eaten a heavy lunch they feel no desire to eat their dinner, and in this case no increase takes place. If they keep their weight at the point reached at the end of the treatment, even a heavy dinner does not bring about an increase of two pounds on the next morning and does not therefore call for any special measures. Most patients are surprised how small their appetite has become and yet how much they can eat without gaining weight. They no longer suffer from an abnormal appetite and feel satisfied with much less food than before. In fact, they are usually disappointed that they cannot manage their first normal meal, which they have been planning for weeks.

Losing more Weight

An ex-patient should never gain more than two pounds without immediately correcting this, but it is equally undesirable that more than two lbs. be lost after treatment, because a greater loss is always achieved at the expense of normal fat. Any normal fat that is lost is invariably regained as soon as more food is taken, and it often happens that this rebound overshoots the upper two lbs. limit.

Trouble After Treatment

Two difficulties may be encountered in the immediate post-treatment period. When a patient has consumed all his abnormal fat or, when after a full course, the injection has temporarily lost its efficacy owing to the body having gradually evolved a counter regulation, the patient at once begins to feel much more hungry and even weak. In spite of repeated warnings, some over-enthusiastic patients do not report this. However, in about two days the fact that they are being undernourished becomes visible in their faces, and treatment is then stopped at once. In such cases — and only in such cases — we allow a very slight increase in the diet, such as an extra apple, 150 grams of meat or two or three extra breadsticks during the three days of dieting after the last injection.

When abnormal fat is no longer being put into circulation either because it has been consumed or because immunity has set in, this is always felt by the patient as sudden, intolerable and constant hunger. In this sense, the HCG method is completely self-limiting. With HCG it is impossible to reduce a patient, however enthusiastic, beyond his normal weight. As soon as no more abnormal fat is being issued, the body starts consuming normal fat, and this is always regained as soon as ordinary feeding is resumed. The patient then finds that the 2-3 lbs. he has lost during the last days of treatment are immediately regained. A meal is skipped and maybe a pound is lost. The next day this pound is regained, in spite of a careful watch over the food intake. In a few days a tearful patient is back in the consulting room, convinced that her case is a failure.

All that is happening is that the essential fat lost at the end of the treatment, owing to the patient's reluctance to report a much greater hunger, is being replaced. The weight at which such a patient must stabilize thus lies 2-3 lbs. higher than the weight reached at the end of the treatment. Once this higher basic level is established, further difficulties in controlling the weight at the new point of stabilization hardly arise.

Beware of Over-Enthusiasm

The other trouble which is frequently encountered immediately after treatment is again due to over-enthusiasm. Some patients cannot believe that they can eat fairly normally without

74

regaining weight. They disregard the advice to eat anything they please except sugar and starch and want to play safe. They try more or less to continue the 500-Calorie diet on which they felt so well during treatment and make only minor variations, such as replacing the meat with an egg, cheese, or a glass of milk. To their horror they find that in spite of this bravura, their weight goes up. So, following instructions, they skip one meager lunch and at night eat only a little salad and drink a pot of unsweetened tea, becoming increasingly hungry and weak. The next morning they find that they have increased yet another pound. They feel terrible, and even the dreaded swelling of their ankles is back. Normally we check our patients one week after they have been eating freely, but these cases return in a few days. Either their eyes are filled with tears or they angrily imply that when we told them to eat normally we were just fooling them.

Protein Deficiency

Here too, the explanation is quite simple. During treatment the patient has been only just above the verge of protein deficiency and has had the advantage of protein being fed back into his system from the breakdown of fatty tissue. Once the treatment is over there is no more HCG in the body and this process no longer takes place. Unless an adequate amount of protein is eaten as soon as the treatment is over, protein deficiency is bound to develop, and this inevitably causes the marked retention of water known as hunger-edema.

The treatment is very simple. The patient is told to eat two eggs for breakfast and a huge steak for lunch and dinner followed by a large helping of cheese and to phone through the weight the next morning. When these instructions are followed a stunned voice is heard to report that two lbs. have vanished overnight, that the ankles are normal but that sleep was disturbed, owing to an extraordinary need to pass large quantities of water. The patient having learned this lesson usually has no further trouble.

Relapses

As a general rule one can say that 60-70% of our cases experience little or no difficulty in holding their weight permanently. Relapses may be due to negligence in the basic rule of daily weighing. Many patients think that this is unnecessary and that they can judge any increase from the fit of their clothes. Some do not carry their scale with them on a journey as it is cumbersome and takes a big bite out of their luggage-allowance when flying. This is a disastrous mistake, because after a course of HCG as much as 10 lbs. can be regained without any noticeable change in the fit of the clothes. The reason for this is that after treatment newly acquired fat is at first evenly distributed and does not show the former preference for certain parts of the body.

Pregnancy or the menopause may annul the effect of a previous treatment. Women who take treatment during the one year after the last menstruation – that is at the onset of the menopause – do just as well as others, but among them the relapse rate is higher until the menopause is fully established. The period of one year after the last menstruation applies only to women who are not being treated with ovarian hormones. If these are taken, the premenopausal period may be indefinitely prolonged.

Late teenage girls who suffer from attacks of compulsive eating have by far the worst record of all as far as relapses are concerned.

Patients who have once taken the treatment never seem to hesitate to come back for another short course as soon as they notice that their weight is once again getting out of hand. They come quite cheerfully and hopefully, assured that they can be helped again. Repeat courses are often even more satisfactory than the first treatment and have the advantage, as do second courses, that the patient already knows that he will feel comfortable throughout.

Plan of a Normal Course

125 I.U. of HCG daily (except during menstruation) until 40 injections have been given.

Until 3rd injection forced feeding.

After 3rd injection, 500 Calorie diet to be continued until 72 hours after the last injection.

For the following 3 weeks, all foods allowed except starch and sugar in any form (careful with very sweet fruit).

After 3 weeks, very gradually add starch in small quantities, always controlled by morning weighing.

CONCLUSION

The HCG + diet method can bring relief to every case of obesity, but the method is not simple. It is very time consuming and requires perfect cooperation between physician and patient. Each case must be handled individually, and the physician must have time to answer questions, allay fears and remove misunderstandings. He must also check the patient daily. When something goes wrong he must at once investigate until he finds the reason for any gain that may have occurred. In most cases it is useless to hand the patient a diet-sheet and let the nurse give him a "shot."

The method involves a highly complex bodily mechanism, and even though our theory may be wrong the physician must make himself some sort of picture of what is actually happening; otherwise he will not be able to deal with such difficulties as may arise during treatment.

I must beg those trying the method for the first time to adhere very strictly to the technique and the interpretations here outlined and thus treat a few hundred cases before embarking on experiments of their own, and until then refrain from introducing innovations, however thrilling they may seem. In a new method, innovations or departures from the original technique can only be usefully evaluated against a substantial background of experience with what is at the moment the orthodox procedure.

I have tried to cover all the problems that come to my mind. Yet a bewildering array of new questions keeps arising, and my interpretations are still fluid. In particular, I have never had an opportunity of conducting the laboratory investigations which are so necessary for a theoretical understanding of clinical observations, and I can only hope that those more fortunately placed will in time be able to fill this gap.

The problems of obesity are perhaps not so dramatic as the problems of cancer, or polio, but they often cause life long suffering. How many promising careers have been ruined by excessive fat; how many lives have been shortened. If some way – however cumbersome – can be found to cope effectively with this universal problem of modern civilized man, our world will be a happier place for countless fellow men and women.

GLOSSARY[9]

ACNE . . . Common skin disease in which pimples, often containing pus, appear on face, neck and shoulders.

ACTH . . . Abbreviation for adrenocorticotrophic hormone. One of the many hormones produced by the anterior lobe of the pituitary gland. ACTH controls the outer part, rind or cortex of the adrenal glands. When ACTH is injected it dramatically relieves arthritic pain, but it has many undesirable side effects, among which is a condition similar to severe obesity. ACTH is now usually replaced by cortisone.

ADRENALIN . . . Hormone produced by the inner part of the Adrenals. Among many other functions, adrenalin is concerned with blood pressure, emotional stress, fear and cold.

ADRENALS . . . Endocrine glands. Small bodies situated atop the kidneys and hence also known as suprarenal glands. The adrenals have an outer rind or cortex which produces vitally important hormones, among which are Cortisone similar substances. The adrenal cortex is controlled by ACTH. The inner part of the adrenals, the medulla, secretes adrenalin and is chiefly controlled by the autonomous nervous system.

ADRENOCORTEX... See adrenals.

AMPHETAMINES . . . Synthetic drugs which reduce the awareness of hunger and stimulate mental activity, rendering sleep impossible. When used for the latter two purposes they are dangerously habit-forming. They do not diminish the body's need for food, but merely suppress the perception of that need. The original drug was known as Benzedrine, from which modern variants such as Dexedrine, Dexamil, and Preludin, etc., have been derived. Amphetamines may help an obese patient to prevent a further increase in weight but are unsatisfactory for reducing, as they do not cure the underlying disorder and as their prolonged use may lead to malnutrition and addiction.

ARTERIOSCLEROSIS . . . Hardening of the arterial wall through the calcification of abnormal deposits of a fatlike substance known as cholesterol.

ASCHHIEIM-ZONDEK . . . Authors of a test by which early pregnancy can be diagnosed by injecting a woman's urine into female mice. The HCG present in pregnancy urine produces certain changes in the vagina of these animals. Many similar tests, using other animals such as rabbits, frogs, etc. have been devised.

ASSIMILATE . . . Absorb digested food from the intestines.

AUTONOMOUS . . . Here used to describe the independent or vegetative nervous system which manages the automatic regulations of the body.

BASAL METABOLISM . . . The body's chemical turnover at complete rest and when fasting. The basal metabolic rate is expressed as the amount of oxygen used up in a given time. The basal metabolic rate (BMR) is controlled by the thyroid gland.

---

[9] Wherever unfamiliar terms are used, they will be found in their respective alphabetical place. The lay reader can therefore make his own cross-reference.

CALORIE . . . The physicist's calorie is the amount of heat required to raise the temperature of 1 cc. of water by 1 degree Centigrade. The dieticiari's Calorie (always written with a capital C) is 1000 times greater. Thus when we speak of a 500 Calorie diet this means that the body is being supplied with as much fuel as would be required to raise the temperature of 500 liters of water by 1 degree Centigrade or 50 liters by 10 degrees. This is quite insufficient to cover the heat and energy requirements of an adult body. In the HCG method the deficit is made up from the abnormal fat-deposits, of which **1 lb. furnishes the body with more than 2000 Calories.** As this is roughly the amount lost every day, a patient under HCG is never short of fuel.

CEREBRAL . . . Of the brain. Cerebral vascular disease is a disorder concerning the blood vessels of the brain, such as cerebral thrombosis or hemorrhage, known as apoplexy or stroke.

CHOLESTEROL . . . A fatlike substance contained in almost every cell of the body. In the blood it exists in two forms, known as free and esterified. The latter form is under certain conditions deposited in the inner lining of the arteries (see arteriosclerosis). No clear and definite relationship between fat intake and cholesterol-level in the blood has yet been established.

CHORIONIC . . . Of the chorion, which is part of the placenta or after-birth. The term chorionic is justly applied to HCG, as this hormone is exclusively produced in the placenta, from where it enters the human mother's blood and is later excreted in her urine.

COMPULSIVE EATING. . . A form of oral gratification with which a repressed sex-instinct is sometimes vicariously relieved. Compulsive eating must not be confused with the real hunger from which most obese patients suffer.

CONGENITAL . . . Any condition which exists at or before birth.

CORONARY ARTERIES . . . Two blood vessels which encircle the heart and supply all the blood required by the heart-muscle.

CORPUS LUTEUM . . . A yellow body which forms in the ovary at the follicle from which an egg has been detached. This body acts as an endocrine gland and plays an important role in menstruation and pregnancy. Its secretion is one of the sex hormones, and it is stimulated by another hormone known as LSH, which stands for luteum stimulating hormones. LSH is produced in the anterior lobe of the pituitary gland. LSH is truly gonadotrophic and must never be confused with HCG, which is a totally different substance, having no direct action on the corpus luteum.

CORTEX . . . Outer covering or rind. The term is applied to the outer part of the adrenals but is also used to describe the gray matter which covers the white matter of the brain.

CORTISONE . . . A synthetic substance which acts like an adrenal hormone. It is today used in the treatment of a large number of illnesses, and several chemical variants have been produced, among which are prednisone and triamcinolone.

CUSHING . . . A great American brain surgeon who described a condition of extreme obesity associated with symptoms of adrenal disorder. Cushing's Syndrome may be caused by organic disease of the pituitary or the adrenal glands but, as was later discovered, it also occurs as a result of excessive ACTH medication.

79

DIENCEPHALON ... A primitive and hence very old part of the brain which lies between and under the two large hemispheres. In man the diencephalon (or hypothalamus) is subordinate to the higher brain or cortex, and yet it ultimately controls all that happens inside the body. It regulates all the endocrine glands, the autonomous nervous system, the turnover of fat and sugar. It seems also to be the seat of the primitive animal instincts and is the relay station at which emotions are translated into bodily reactions.

DIURETIC. .. Any substance that increases the flow of urine.

DYSFUNCTION ... Abnormal functioning of any organ, be this excessive, deficient or in any way altered.

EDEMA ... An abnormal accumulation of water in the tissues.

ELECTROCARDIOGRAM ... Tracing of electric phenomena taking place in the heart during each beat. The tracing provides information about the condition and working of the heart which is not otherwise obtainable.

ENDOCRINE ... We distinguish endocrine and exocrine glands. The former produce hormones, chemical regulators, which they secrete directly into the blood circulation in the gland and from where they are carried all over the body. Examples of endocrine glands are the pituitary, the thyroid and the adrenals. Exocrine glands produce a visible secretion such as saliva, sweat, urine. There are also glands which are endocrine and exocrine. Examples are the testicles, the prostate and the pancreas, which produces the hormone insulin and digestive ferments which flow from the gland into the intestinal tract. Endocrine glands are closely inter dependent of each other, they are linked to the autonomous nervous system and the diencephalon presides over this whole incredibly complex regulatory system.

EMACIATED ... Grossly undernourished.

EUPHORIA ... A feeling of particular physical and mental well being.

FERAL ... Wild, unrestrained.

FIBROID ... Any benign new growth of connective tissue. When such a tumor originates from a muscle, it is known as a myoma. The most common seat of myomas is the uterus.

FOLLICLE ... Any small bodily cyst or sac containing a liquid. Here the term applies to the ovarian cyst in which the egg is formed. The egg is expelled when a ripe follicle bursts and this is known as ovulation (see corpus luteum).

FSH ... Abbreviation for follicle-stimulating hormone. FSH is another (see corpus luteum) anterior pituitary hormone which acts directly on the ovarian follicle and is therefore correctly called a gonadotrophin.

GLANDS ... See endocrine.

GONADOTROPHIN ... See corpus luteum, follicle and FSH. Gonadotrophic literally means sex gland-directed. FSH, LSH and the equivalent hormones in the male, all produced in the anterior lobe of the pituitary gland, are true gonadotrophins. Unfortunately and confusingly, the term gonadotrophin has also been applied to the placental hormone of pregnancy known as human chorionic gonadotrophin (HCG). This hormone acts on the diencephalon and can only indirectly influence the sex-glands via the anterior lobe of the pituitary.

80

HCG . . . Abbreviation for human chorionic gonadotrophin

HORMONES . . . See endocrine.

HYPERTENSION . . . High blood pressure.

HYPOGLYCEMIA . . . A condition in which the blood sugar is below normal. It can be relieved by eating sugar.

HYPOPHYSIS . . . Another name for the pituitary gland.

HYPOTHESIS. . . A tentative explanation or speculation on how observed facts and isolated scientific data can be brought into an intellectually satisfying relationship of cause and effect. Hypotheses are useful for directing further research, but they are not necessarily an exposition of what is believed to be the truth. Before a hypothesis can advance to the dignity of a theory or a law, it must be confirmed by all future research. As soon as research turns up data which no longer fit the hypothesis, it is immediately abandoned for a better one.

LSH . . . See corpus luteum.

METABOLISM . . . See basal metabolism.

MIGRAINE. . . Severe half-sided headache often associated with vomiting.

MUCOID . . . Slime-like.

MYOCARDIUM . . . The heart-muscle.

MYOMA . . . See fibroid.

MYXEDEMA. . . Accumulation of a mucoid substance in the tissues which occurs in cases of severe primary thyroid deficiency.

NEOLITHIC . . . In the history of human culture we distinguish the Early Stone Age or Paleolithic, the Middle Stone Age or Mesolithic and the New Stone Age or Neolithic period. The Neolithic period started about 8000 years ago when the first attempts at agriculture, pottery and animal domestication made at the end of the Mesolithic period suddenly began to develop rapidly along the road that led to modern civilization.

NORMAL SALINE . . . A low concentration of salt in water equal to the salinity of body fluids.

PHLEBITIS. . . An inflammation of the veins. When a blood-clot forms at the site of the inflammation, we speak of thrombophlebitis.

PITUITARY . . . A very complex endocrine gland which lies at the base of the skull, consisting chiefly of an anterior and a posterior lobe. The pituitary is controlled by the diencephalon, which regulates the anterior lobe by means of hormones which reach it through small blood vessels. The posterior lobe is controlled by nerves which run from the diencephalon into this part of the gland. The anterior lobe secretes many hormones, among which are those that regulate other glands such as the thyroid, the adrenals and the sex glands.

PLACENTA . . . The after-birth. In women, a large and highly complex organ through which the child in the womb receives its nourishment from the mother's body. It is the organ in which HCG is manufactured and then given off into the mother's blood.

PROTEIN ... The living substance in plant and animal cells. Herbivorous animals can thrive on plant protein alone, but man must have some protein of animal origin (milk, eggs or flesh) to live healthily. When insufficient protein is eaten, the body retains water.

PSORIASIS ... A skin disease which produces scaly patches. These tend to disappear during pregnancy and during the treatment of obesity by the HCG method.

RENAL ... Of the kidney.

RESERPINE ... An Indian drug extensively used in the treatment of high blood pressure and some forms of mental disorder.

RETENTION ENEMA ... The slow infusion of a liquid into the rectum, from where it is absorbed and not evacuated.

SACRUM ... A fusion of the lower vertebrate into the large bony mass to which the pelvis is attached.

SEDIMENTATION RATE ... The speed at which a suspension of red blood cells settles out. A rapid settling out is called a high sedimentation rate and may be indicative of a large number of bodily disorders of pregnancy.

SEXUAL SELECTION ... A sexual preference for individuals which show certain traits. If this preference or selection goes on generation after generation, more and more individuals showing the trait will appear among the general population. The natural environment has little or nothing to do with this process. Sexual selection therefore differs from natural selection, to which modern man is no longer subject because he changes his environment rather than let the environment change him.

STRIATION ... Tearing of the lower layers of the skin owing to rapid stretching in obesity or during pregnancy. When first formed striae are dark reddish lines which later change into white scars.

SUPRARENAL GLANDS ... See adrenals.

SYNDROME ... A group of symptoms which in their association are characteristic of a particular disorder.

THROMBOPHLEBITIS ... See phlebitis.

THROMBUS ... A blood-clot in a blood-vessel.

TRIAMCINOLONE ... A modern derivative of cortisone.

URIC ACID ... A product of incomplete protein-breakdown or utilization in the body. When uric acid becomes deposited in the gristle of the joints we speak of gout.

VARICOSE ULCERS ... Chronic ulceration above the ankles due to varicose veins which interfere with the normal blood circulation in the affected areas.

VEGETATIVE ... See autonomous.

VERTEBRATE ... Any animal that has a back-bone.

Literary References to the Use of
Chorionic Gonadotrophin
In Obesity

THE LANCET

Nov. 6, 1954	Article	Simeons
Nov. 15, 1958	Letter to Editor	Simeons
July 29, 1961	Letter to Editor	Lebon
Dec. 9, 1961	Article	Carne
Dec. 9, 1961	Letter to Editor	Kalina
Jan. 6, 1962	Letter to Editor	Simeons
Nov. 26, 1966	Letter to Editor	Lebon

THE JOURNAL OF THE AMERICAN GERIATRIC SOCIETY

Jan. 1956	Article	Simeons
Oct. 1964	Article	Harris & Warsaw
Feb. 1966	Article	Lebon

THE AMERICAN JOURNAL OF CLINICAL NUTRITION

Sept.-Oct. 1959	Article	Sohar
March 1963	Article	Craig et al.
Sept. 1963	Letter to Editor	Simeons
March 1964	Article	Frank
Sept. 1964	Letter to Editor	Simeons
Feb. 1965	Letter to Editor	Hutton
June 1969	Editorial	Albrink
June 1969	Special Article	Gusman

THE JOURNAL OF PLASTIC SURGERY (British)

April 1962	Article	Lebon

THE SOUTH AFRICAN MEDICAL JOURNAL

Feb 1963	Article	Politzer, Berson & Flaks

BOOKS

A.T.W. SIMEONS
**POUNDS AND INCHES Privately printed: obtainable only from
A.T.W. Simeons, Salvator Mundi International Hospital, Rome,
Italy**
**VETSUCHT (Netherlands Edition) Wetenschappelijke Uitgeverij,
N.V. Amsterdam**
MAN'S PRESUMPTUOUS BRAIN Longman's, Green, London
 E.P. Dutton, New York (hardback)
 Dutton Paperbacks, New York

Audio File Link

To listen to the Pounds and Inches: A New Approach to Obesity manuscript on your MP3 player, just sign up to download the audio file from this link:
http://tinyurl.com/AudioSignup

Pounds and Inches Pocket Reference

Phase 1

HCG Checklist

This plan works much better if you plan and prepare. I used this list to ensure that I did not forget anything. You may print this list out and check off the items with a pen. The book referenced in this checklist is the original unabridged book *HCG Diet Made Simple: Your Step-By-Step Guide Beyond Pounds and Inches*, not this Pocket Reference book, which is not intended to be a detailed guide to the HCG Diet.

☐   1.   Read the original unabridged book *HCG Diet Made Simple: Your Step-By-Step Guide Beyond Pounds and Inches* in its entirety.

☐   2.   Take a "before" picture of yourself. Yes, it is humbling, but you will be glad you did later, when it is time for a side by side comparison of before and after.

☐   3.   Take your "before" measurements. Again, you will be happy that you did.

☐   4.   Read Dr. Simeons' "Pounds and Inches."

☐   5.   Apply to join the HCG Diet Made Simple support group by sending an email to: HCGDietMadeSimple-subscribe@yahoogroups.com or scanning this code with your Smartphone and clicking "Join This Group":

☐   6.   Take stock of your personal readiness state.

Answer the following questions for yourself:

☐   o   Can you commit to staying on the program for the time needed?

☐   o   How easily can you fit the program into your lifestyle?

☐   o   What opposition will you have from family and friends?

☐   o   What support will you have from family and friends?

☐   o   Will you have the support and help of your doctor?

☐   o   Will you be confident enough to do the program on your own, or do you need to use a clinic to provide you with meds and support?

☐   o   Do you have the financial means to purchase the needed supplies?

☐   o   Do you have the time needed to complete at least one round?

☐   o   Are you ready to change your life?

☐   7. Decide if you need a new scale to weigh your body.

☐   8. Read "Pounds and Inches" AGAIN!!!

☐   9. Approach your doctor about the protocol, if you choose to do so.

☐   10. Determine whether your doctor will be supportive or actually prescribe the hCG for you.

☐   11. If your doctor will not support you, review the Clinics section of the book.

☐   12. Decide whether to use a clinic or go it on your own.

☐   13. Choose a clinic, if needed.

☐   14. If doing this without a clinic or physician:

☐   o   Decide whether to do Subcutaneous or Intramuscular injections OR use a sublingual mixture.

☐   o   Determine how much hCG you will need to lose the weight you want.

- [ ]   1. What dosage will you take?
- [ ]   2. How many rounds do you need to do?
- [ ]   3. Will other family or friends be doing the program with you?
- [ ]   ○ Review the hCG suppliers section of the book and decide where to order hCG.
- [ ]   ○ Order hCG.
- [ ]   ○ Review the book sections for your chosen administration method and determine what supplies for giving injections or mixing sublingual that you need to purchase.
- [ ]   ○ Order supplies.
- [ ] 15. Plan your program by deciding your schedule for Phases and rounds, considering holidays, vacations, and special events.
- [ ] 16. If necessary, buy scales for weighing yourself and your food.
- [ ] 17. Become educated about Cleanses for Phase 1.
- [ ] 18. Purchase and use cleanses and other Phase I options, if you choose to do so.
- [ ] 19. Become educated about organic food.
- [ ] 20. Determine sources for organic food, if you choose to do so.
- [ ] 21. Begin purchasing and eating organic, if you choose to do so.
- [ ] 22. Visit **www.hcgdieterstore.com** to see some products that can be used on the protocol.
- [ ] 23. Change to protocol-compliant personal care products, if you choose to do so.
- [ ] 24. Mentally prepare for Phase 2.
- [ ] 25. Review the section in the book on the Recipes for the diet plan and food preparation.
- [ ] 26. Plan your Phase 2 meals for the first week using the Meal Planning Auto Calorie Calculator Spreadsheet.

- [ ] 27. Set interim goals for yourself so that you can celebrate your success along the way.
- [ ] 28. If doing this on your own, on the first day of Phase 2, mix the hCG and store it properly.
- [ ] 29. Begin your hCG administration method of choice.
- [ ] 30. Decide how to handle other people while on the diet.
- [ ] 31. Weigh yourself each day and record the weight in the Pounds and Inches Tracking Spreadsheet.
- [ ] 32. Load TO CAPACITY with lots of fats for the first two days of hCG administration.
- [ ] 33. Begin the 500 calorie food plan (VLCD) on day three.
- [ ] 34. Record your food each day, to be used for analysis purposes later, if not reducing weight.
- [ ] 35. If continuing Phase 2 past 23 days, skip hCG one day a week, but continue 500 calories on that day.
- [ ] 36. If you remain at the same weight for four days, you may do an apple day, as described on pages 68-69 of "Pounds and Inches".
- [ ] 37. Begin your preparation mentally for Phase 3.
- [ ] 38. One week before discontinuation of hCG, begin planning Phase 3 meals with no refined sugar or starch. Do NOT limit fat, salt, or anything else. Plan in particular for much more protein, as you are on the verge of protein deficiency when beginning Phase 3.
- [ ] 39. Review the Phase 3 lists of sugars and starches.
- [ ] 40. Record your weight on your last injection or sublingual dose day. This is your LIW.
- [ ] 41. Continue 500 calories for 72 hours after the last injection. You may continue to lose on these days.
- [ ] 42. Review the sample Phase 3 menu. Do NOT continue 500 calories after this. It is very important to eat MUCH more food and in particular, protein, for three weeks. Eat foods that were not allowed in Phase 2, but still do not have refined sugar or

starch. Do NOT be afraid of fat. Use full-fat products, NOT low-fat or non-fat.

☐ 43. Continue to weigh yourself daily in Phase 3.

☐ 44. If you weigh more than 2 pounds over your last injection weight or last sublingual dose weight on any day, you must do a steak day on that day as described on pages 92-93 of "Pounds and Inches". Do not wait. Do it that day.

☐ 45. If you suspect that you have edema (water retention) caused by insufficient protein, do the eggs-steak-cheese day as described on page 96 of "Pounds and Inches".

☐ 46. After completing three weeks of no refined sugar or starches, you may proceed to Phase 4, gradually adding sugars and starches. Dr. Simeons requires three weeks of Phase 4 before beginning your second round of Phase 2, if needed. If you have reached your goal weight, CELEBRATE!!!

For all of the details of all of these steps, the unabridged book *HCG Diet Made Simple: Your Step-by-Step Guide Beyond Pounds and Inches* by the same author contains the complete details surrounding all of these steps. This Pocket Reference does not.

Day-by-Day on HCG

These handy charts show what you are doing on each day of a round of HCG.

Short Round (skipping one day a week not required)

23 injections (or doses), if NOT skipping one day a week, assuming that injections are given in the morning

Day	Protocol Followed	Injections	Effective Injections
1	Load + hCG	1	
2	Load + hCG	2	
3	VLCD + hCG	3	
4	VLCD + hCG	4	1
5	VLCD + hCG	5	2
6	VLCD + hCG	6	3
7	VLCD + hCG	7	4
8	VLCD + hCG	8	5
9	VLCD + hCG	9	6
10	VLCD + hCG	10	7
11	VLCD + hCG	11	8
12	VLCD + hCG	12	9
13	VLCD + hCG	13	10
14	VLCD + hCG	14	11
15	VLCD + hCG	15	12
16	VLCD + hCG	16	13
17	VLCD + hCG	17	14
18	VLCD + hCG	18	15
19	VLCD + hCG	19	16

Day	Protocol Followed	Injections	Effective Injections
20	VLCD + hCG	20	17
21	VLCD + hCG	21	18
22	VLCD + hCG	22	19
23	VLCD + hCG	23	20
24	VLCD	24	
25	VLCD	25	
26	Phase 3		

Short Round if skipping one day a week

23 injections (or doses), if skipping one day a week (not required for a short round), assuming that injections are given in the morning

Day	Protocol Followed	Injections	Effective Injections
1	Load + hCG	1	
2	Load + hCG	2	
3	VLCD + hCG	3	
4	VLCD + hCG	4	1
5	VLCD + hCG	5	2
6	VLCD + hCG	6	3
7	VLCD		
8	VLCD + hCG	7	4
9	VLCD + hCG	8	5
10	VLCD + hCG	9	6
11	VLCD + hCG	10	7
12	VLCD + hCG	11	8

Day	Protocol Followed	Injections	Effective Injections
13	VLCD + hCG	12	9
14	VLCD		
15	VLCD + hCG	13	10
16	VLCD + hCG	14	11
17	VLCD + hCG	15	12
18	VLCD + hCG	16	13
19	VLCD + hCG	17	14
20	VLCD + hCG	18	15
21	VLCD		
22	VLCD + hCG	19	16
23	VLCD + hCG	20	17
24	VLCD + hCG	21	18
25	VLCD + hCG	22	19
26	VLCD + hCG	23	20
27	VLCD		
28	VLCD		
29	Phase 3		

Long Round, skipping one day a week as required

40 injections (or doses), skipping one day a week as required, assuming that injections are given in the morning

Day	Protocol Followed	Injections	Effective Injections
1	Load + hCG	1	
2	Load + hCG	2	
3	VLCD + hCG	3	

Day	Protocol Followed	Injections	Effective Injections
4	VLCD + hCG	4	1
5	VLCD + hCG	5	2
6	VLCD + hCG	6	3
7	VLCD		
8	VLCD + hCG	7	4
9	VLCD + hCG	8	5
10	VLCD + hCG	9	6
11	VLCD + hCG	10	7
12	VLCD + hCG	11	8
13	VLCD + hCG	12	9
14	VLCD		
15	VLCD + hCG	13	10
16	VLCD + hCG	14	11
17	VLCD + hCG	15	12
18	VLCD + hCG	16	13
19	VLCD + hCG	17	14
20	VLCD + hCG	18	15
21	VLCD		
22	VLCD + hCG	19	16
23	VLCD + hCG	20	17
24	VLCD + hCG	21	18
25	VLCD + hCG	22	19
26	VLCD + hCG	23	20

Day	Protocol Followed	Injections	Effective Injections
27	VLCD + hCG	24	21
28	VLCD		
29	VLCD + hCG	25	22
30	VLCD + hCG	26	23
31	VLCD + hCG	27	24
32	VLCD + hCG	28	25
33	VLCD + hCG	29	26
34	VLCD + hCG	30	27
35	VLCD		
36	VLCD + hCG	31	28
37	VLCD + hCG	32	29
38	VLCD + hCG	33	30
39	VLCD + hCG	34	31
40	VLCD + hCG	35	32
41	VLCD + hCG	36	33
42	VLCD		
43	VLCD + hCG	37	34
44	VLCD + hCG	38	35
45	VLCD + hCG	39	36
46	VLCD + hCG	40	37
47	VLCD		
48	VLCD		
49	Phase 3		

Phase 2

Ordering Information

hCG is sold under many brand names and is provided by pharmaceutical companies such as Schering, Serono, Squib, Ferring, Organon, Parke-Davis, Wyeth Ayerst, Steris, Fujisawa, and others. Brands of hCG from India would be Corion or Profasi made by Serono. Pregnyl, made by Organon is ordered from Europe/Greece. Lepori, made by Farma-Lepori, is from Spain. IBSA Choriomon is NOT made in Mexico, but is available at pharmacies there. It is from Switzerland. If you are in a country that allows you to buy hCG over the counter, you need to know the brand names in order to ask for it at a pharmacy.

Here is a handy table listing most of the names for hCG:

Brand Name	IU	Manufacturer
APL (US, SA)	5000, 10000 or 20000 IU	Wyeth-Ayerst
Abraxis		Abraxis Pharmaceutical Products (APP)
Antuitrin S		Parke-Davis
Biogonadyl (PL)	500 or 2000 IU	Biomed
Chorionic Gonadotropin		Steris or Fujisawa
Choragon (G)	1500 or 5000 IU	Ferring Pharmaceuticals
Chorex-5; Chorex-10;Chorex (US)	5000 or 10000 IU	Hyrex
Chorigon		
Choriolife		Life Medicare
Choriolutin (G)		
Choriomon	5000 IU	IBSA, Switzerland
Choron 10 (US)	1000 or 10000 IU	Forest
Chorvlon (A)		
Corgonject		
Corion		Win Medicare
Dinaron		

Brand Name	IU	Manufacturer
Ekluton (G)		
Endocorion		
Fertigyn		Sun Pharmaceuticals (Inca Division)
Follutein		Squib
G. Chor. "Endo" (FR)	500, 1500 or 5000 IU	Organon
Gestyl (BG)	1000 IU	Organon
Glukor (US)		
Gonacor		
Gonadatrophon (GB)	500,1000 or 500 IU	Paines & Byrne
Gonadotraphon LH (I)	1000, 2000 or 5000 IU	Amsa
Gonadotropyl-C (MX/FR)	5000 IU	Roussel
Gonakor (MX)	2500 IU	Sanfer
Gonic (US)	1000 IU	Roberts
Harvatropin (US)		
HCG (US)	5000 or 10000 IU	Pharmed or Steris
HCG Lepori (ES)	500, 1000 or 2500 IU	Lepori
Hucog		Bharat Serum & Vaccines
LG IVF – C		LG Life Sciences
Life		Solvay Pharma
Neogonadil Bruco		
Novarel®		Ferring Pharmaceuticals
Ovidac		Zydus Cadila
Ovidrel recombinant hCG (r-hCG)		Serono (division of Merck)
Ovogest (G)		
Ovo-Gonadon (G)		
Ovutrig – HP		VHB Life Sciences
Physex (DK,NO)	1500 or 3000 IU	Leo
Physex Leo (ES)	500,1500 or 5000 IU	Leo

Brand Name	IU	Manufacturer
Praedyn (CZ)	1500 or 3000 IU	Leciva
Predalon (G)	500 or 5000 IU	Organon
Pregnesin (G,CZ)	1000, 2500 or 5000 IU	Serono
Pregnyl		Organon India (Infar)
Pregnyl (A,B,CH,GB,BG,GR,I,NL,PL,S,FI,YU,CZ,NO,HU)	5000 IU	Organon
Pregnyl (BG)	100 IU	Organon
Pregnyl (US)	10000 IU	Organon
Primogonyl (G,CH,YU,CZ)	5000 IU	Schering
Profasi (A,B,CH,DK,HU,GB,GR,S,FR,NL,NO,MX)	2000 or 5000 IU	Serono Serum International
Profasi (CH,B,MX,S,FI,GB,NO,NL)	10000 IU	Serono
Profasi (CH,GB,MX,HU,FR)	500 IU	Serono
Profasi (FR)	1500 IU	Serono
Profasi (HU,NL,MX)	1000 IU	Serono
Provigil hCG b		Maneesh Pharmaceuticals
Pubergen		Uni – Sankyo
Rochoric (US)		
ZY – HCG		Zydus Cadila (Biogen Division)

Sources of HCG

Sources of hCG	Description	Cost	Website / Payment Accepted	Comments
Escrow Refills Do not order premixed. Also has mixing kits.	1 x 2000 IU 3 x 2000 IU 5 x 2000 IU 1 x 5000 IU 3 x 5000 IU 5 x 5000 IU 10 x 5000 IU	$19.94 $48.44 $76.94 $30.39 $80.74 $132.04 $243.19 $25 s&h	http://tinyurl.com/hcglink 14 Visa, Check/ Money Orders Can use a prepaid international credit card bought from a drugstore if you don't have a Visa.	**IMPORTANT:** To enter the site, just type in the invitation code CID292127 and click Continue to get $30 off of your first order. You MUST order when entering the site the FIRST time, or you can't get back in with ANY code without using another computer or browser. Delivery: 2 weeks
Anabolic Pharmacy	1 x 1500 IU 1 x 5000 IU 5 x 5000 IU	$21.12 $30.36 $139.92 $18 s&h	http://tinyurl.com/hcglink 4 Visa/MasterCard/Amex	Delivery: 12-30 working days Will ship to Canada Does NOT reship if confiscated
Eurobolic	1 x 1500 IU 3 x 5000 IU	$38.17 $98.71 $20 s&h	http://tinyurl.com/hcglink 13 Western Union Money Transfer, Direct Bank Transfer, and MoneyGram	Delivery: 8 to 15 days
Reliable Rx	1 x 2000 IU 1 x 5000 IU	$16.00 $19.00 $20 s&h	http://tinyurl.com/hcglink 9	Delivery: 10 working days.
Sport Pharma	1 x 1500 IU 1 x 2000 IU 1 x 5000 IU	$18.62 $19.95 $29.26 $20 s&h	http://tinyurl.com/hcglink 10 Visa/MasterCard/Western Union	Delivery: 8 to 18 days. Hands your order off to a drop-shipper and therefore canNOT verify whether the order was shipped or give tracking information.
Sustanon Deca	1 x 1500 IU 1 x 5000 IU	$27.64 $35.53 $20 s&h	http://tinyurl.com/hcglink 11 Western Union Money Transfer, Direct Bank Transfer, and MoneyGram	Delivery: 10 to 12 days.
Canada Pharmacy	1 x 2000 IU 1 x 5000 IU	$38.00 $44.00 $10 s&h	http://tinyurl.com/hcglink 15 Visa/MasterCard/PayPal	Delivery: 6 to 20 days.

Sources of Injection/Sublingual Supplies

Suppliers of Injection/ Sublingual Supplies, NOT HCG	Description	Cost	Website Address / Forms of Payment Accepted	Comments
HCG Supplies	hCG-specific Kits with: syringes, needles, alcohol pads, vials, larger syringes for mixing.	Varies by kit. Priority Mail is FREE	http://tinyurl.com/hcgsupplies Amex/Visa/MasterCard	Most convenient way to get started. Fast delivery. Great customer service, very knowledgeable.
HCG Coach Kits	Sublingual or injection kits Coaching	Varies by kit	http://tinyurl.com/supplies4 Click the second link that displays and use code "Harmony" in the Notes box for $5 off any order over $25.00.	Fast delivery. Great customer service, very knowledgeable
Michele's Discount Supplies	Both mixing kits and single items	Varies	http://tinyurl.com/supplies7	Fast delivery. Great customer service, very knowledgeable
AndroUSA	Needles, syringes, vials, bacteriostatic water	Varies $9.85 s&h	http://tinyurl.com/supplies1 Amex/Discover/Visa/ MasterCard	Fast delivery. Great customer service, very knowledgeable.
GPZ Services	Injection supplies	Varies	http://tinyurl.com/supplies2 Amex/Discover/Visa/ MasterCard	Fast delivery.
Medlab Supply	Syringes, needles, vials, bacteriostatic water	Varies	http://tinyurl.com/supplies3 Amex/Discover/Visa/ MasterCard/PayPal/West ern Union	Fast delivery. E- GPZ mail notification of shipment and tracking.

HCG Coaching

Only two hCG coaches make up the list of those I trust to guide people through the diet personally. That's because I want to only recommend those that I know personally to be the best.

Shalom Shick

Shalom is a Student ND (Naturopathic Doctor) with Trinity College of Natural Health. She can be contacted at www.HCGCoach.com. If you place an order, just enter "Harmony" into the coupon code to get 5% off.

Vicky Rowe

Vicky is a Board Certified Nutritional Counseling and Weight Loss Coach, CHHP, CHT, AADP. Contact her at:

www.SatoriHolisticHealth.com or at 919-554-4625 if you prefer to call.

Quick Clinic Comparison Chart

Differences /Clinics	Clinical HCG	GHI	Trans-Form-ations	Releana
Cost of hCG	$217 for the hCG and all supplies, with $38 charge for shipping from the pharmacy. If you don't want to do injections, they sell the hCG nasal spray for $227.	Premixed injections, $305 for 6 weeks	$50 a week for hCG and appetite suppressants. $25 a week for hCG only	Premixed Sublingual, $250 for 30 days
Cost of Required Labs	Unknown	$250 labs and $200 doc review	$130	Unknown
Freeze hCG?	No	Yes	No, they don't even state to refrigerate.	No, but they do state to refrigerate.

Quick Program Comparison Chart

Differences /Programs	Simeons	Clinical HCG	GHI	Trans- form- ations	Releana
Calories per day allowed	500	500	No food plan	800.	Doctor-dependent
Grissini /Melba	Yes	Yes	Yes	Yes	No
Oranges	Yes	Yes	Yes	Yes	Yes
Shellfish	Yes	Yes	Yes	Yes	Yes
Broccoli/ Cauliflower/ Zucchini	No	No	Yes	Yes	Yes
Mix Vegetables	No	No	Yes	Yes	Yes
Organic	No	No	No	No	No
Cleanses	No	No	No	No	No
Skip a Day	Yes	Yes	No	Yes, 2	No
Daily Dose	125IU	125IU	250IU	125IU	166IU x2
Stop During Period	Yes	Yes	Yes	No	No
Administra-tion method	IM injection	IM injection	SC/SQ injection	SC/SQ injection	Sublingual
Per Course Loss Limit	34 lbs or 40 lbs if obese	34 lbs or 40 lbs if obese	None	None	None
Per Course Dose Limit	40 injections	40 doses	40 doses	40 doses	None
Break length	6 weeks 8 weeks 12 wks, etc.	6 weeks 8 weeks 12 wks, etc.	2 weeks	3 weeks	None

Shopping Guide for Phase 2

Shopping List

The allowed food list from Pounds and Inches is:

BREAKFAST: Tea or coffee in any quantity without sugar. Only one tablespoonful of milk allowed in 24 hours. Saccharin or other sweeteners may be used. [Author's note: I only recommend stevia and erythritol sweeteners during the diet, as they are zero-glycemic.]

LUNCH:

1. 100 grams of veal, beef, chicken breast, fresh white fish, lobster, crab, or shrimp. All visible fat must be carefully removed before cooking, and the meat must be weighed raw. It must be boiled or grilled without additional fat. Salmon, eel, tuna, herring, dried or pickled fish are not allowed. The chicken breast must be removed raw from the bird.
2. One type of vegetable only to be chosen from the following: spinach, chard, chicory, beet-greens, green salad, tomatoes, celery, fennel, onions, red radishes, cucumbers, asparagus, cabbage.
3. One breadstick (grissino) or one Melba toast.
4. An apple or an orange or a handful of strawberries or one-half grapefruit.

DINNER: The same four choices as lunch.

Occasional Alternative Sources of Protein

"Very occasionally we allow egg – boiled, poached or raw – to patients who develop an aversion to meat, but in this case they must add the white of three eggs to the one they eat whole. In countries where cottage cheese made from skimmed milk is available 100 grams may occasionally be used instead of the meat, but no other cheeses are allowed." Pounds and Inches, page 63

What's the difference between "all natural" and "organic"?

All natural refers to no additives and *is based on testimony of the producer*. **Organic** means the product comes from at least 90% organic ingredients, but **100% organic** means 100% of the ingredients are organic. **Certified organic** must come from animals whose parents were certified raised organic and raised from birth on organic land. They must be fed organic crops. The land cannot have been sprayed with pesticides, herbicides, fungicides, or synthetic fertilizers for a minimum of 3 years prior to certification. No animal byproducts may be fed to certified organic animals. No genetically engineered organisms (GMOs) may be used in feed or the animals. The product to be certified must be documented from birth to purchaser for traceability and verification. Antibiotics cannot be used in organic meat.

What's the difference between the different types of meat?

I did some research on meat and spoke to my butcher. This is the information that I received.

o **Regular beef** is usually kept very contained and fed hormones, antibiotics and supplements as well as grains, and ground-up animal by-products. Most of the animal by-products are from animals that were sick and not fit for human consumption. (Cows are not supposed to eat meat!!) Since the animals are contained, they don't get any exercise and toxins aren't able to be released from their bodies.

o Some animals are given all the hormones, antibiotics, and supplements as well as the grains and animal by-products but allowed time to roam free. In my area this is called **free-range meat**.

o **All natural beef** starts its life as regular beef but is allowed to roam free in the fields and is not given any hormones, antibiotics, or supplements for at least the last few months of its life. It is still fed grains. It's better than regular beef.

o **Organic beef** is never given any hormones, antibiotics, supplements, etc. Neither have their parents. They are never given any feed that is grown with the use of pesticides or chemical fertilizers. (The ground can't have been sprayed for at least 3 years where the feed is grown.) The animals are treated by natural methods if they become ill. If that doesn't work and the farmer needs to use an injection to cure the animal, it is labeled and sold as regular beef. These animals are free to roam their entire lives. They are also fed grains.

o **Grass fed only organic beef** is never fed grains. They eat in the fields and are fed hay when weather doesn't permit them to free graze. The proven benefits of eating "Grass-Only Beef" include: less fat, fewer calories, more Omega-3 fatty acids, a healthier ratio of Omega-6 to Omega-3 fatty acids, more Conjugated Linoleic Acid (CLA), more Vitamin E and higher levels of beta-carotene. This is the best meat.

Leanest Beef Cuts	Leanest Veal Cuts
Top Round (Inside Round Steak)	Leg Cutlet
Eye of Round	Blade Steak
Round Tip or Bottom Round	Rib Roast
Shank or Arm	Shoulder Steak
Sirloin Steak	Loin Chop
Rump Roast	
Top Loin	
T-Bone	
Tenderloin or Filet	

What are considered to be the white fish that ARE allowed in Phase 2?

Ayr, Catfish, Cod, Coley, Flounder, Flying fish, Haddock, Hake, Halibut, Hoki, John dory, Kalabasu, Ling, Monk fish, Parrot fish, Plaice, Pollack, Pomfret, Red & grey mullet, Red fish, Red Snapper, Rohu, Rock Salmon/Dogfish, Sea bass, Sea bream, Shark, Skate, Sole, Tilapia, Turbot, and Whiting Cod

What are considered to be fatty fish that ARE NOT allowed in Phase 2?

Anchovies, Bloater, Cacha, Carp, Eel, Herring, Hilsa, Jack fish, Katla, Kipper, Mackerel, Orange roughy, Pangas, Pilchards, Salmon, Sardines, Sprats, Swordfish, Trout, Tuna, and Whitebate

Nutritive Oils to Avoid in Lotions and Cosmetics

Glycerin and pure essential oils such as lavender are fine, as they are non-nutritive in a food sense; but any oil associated with a food, such as lemon seed or other seeds, lanolin, coconut, shea butter, palm, cocoa, olive, sunflower, almond, or safflower oils will be absorbed by the skin and recognized by the body as food. You'd be surprised how many modern products contain those things.

Sample Menus

Phase 2 Sample Menu 1

Breakfast: ½ grapefruit

Coffee with vanilla stevia and 1 T milk

Lunch: 3.5 oz grilled chicken with lettuce salad using herbs, salt, and apple cider vinegar

Afternoon snack: 6 strawberries

Dinner: 6 grilled shrimp with garlic salt and Cajun spices with steamed spinach seasoned with lemon juice

Phase 2 Sample Menu 2

Breakfast: Orange	62 calories
Snack: Raw Cabbage with vinegar in a slaw	35 calories
Lunch: 3.5 ounces Chicken sautéed with Cabbage	155 calories
Snack: Tomato sliced with salt and pepper	36 calories
Dinner: 3.5 ounces Chicken sautéed with Tomato and Cajun seasoning	141 calories
Snack: Apple	67 calories
Total:	496 calories

Phase 2 Sample Menu 3

Lunch: Pink Lady Apple, Roasted Tomatoes, 3.5 oz White Fish

Dinner: Honeycrisp Apple, Romaine Lettuce, 3.5 oz Ground Sirloin

Phase 2 Sample Menu 4

Breakfast: Coffee with 1 T milk and Cinnamon Liquid Stevia

Snack: ½ grapefruit

Lunch: Shrimp with salad and Melba toast

Dinner: Chicken and asparagus with grissini breadstick

Snack: Baked Apple with Cinnamon Liquid Stevia

Calorie Calculator and Food Record

Day/Date			
Food Item	**Calories/Oz**	**Oz eaten**	**Calories**
Fruit (serving)			
Apple, raw (1 whole)	15		
Grapefruit, raw (1/2 only)	9		
Orange, raw (1 whole)	13		
Strawberries, raw (handful)	9		
Vegetable			
Asparagus, raw	6		
Beet Greens	6		
Cabbage	7		
Celery	4		
Chard	7		
Chicory	7		
Cucumber	3		
Fennel	9		
Lettuce, Romaine	5		
Lettuce, Iceburg	4		
Onion, bulb raw	12		
Onion, green	9		
Radish	5		
Spinach	7		
Tomatoes, raw	5		
Protein (3.5 ounces per meal)			
Catfish/Crab	27		
Chicken Breast	31		
Flounder/Sole	26		
Haddock	25		
Halibut	31		
Hamburger 85% lean	60		
Hamburger 90% Lean	50		
Hamburger 95% Lean	38		
Lobster	28		
Prawn	30		
Red Snapper	28		
Steak, sirloin	37		
Shrimp, shelled	30		
Tilapia	27		
Veal, top round	38		
Alternative Protein			
Cottage Cheese, nonfat (4 oz)	80 total		
Eggs (1 whole + 3 whites)	129 Total		
Starch			
Melba or Grissini (1 per meal)	20 each		
Lemon Juice-Wedge	1		
DAILY CALORIE TOTAL			
CALORIES LEFT			

Pounds and Inches Mixing Calculator

Ampoule Size (IU)	Desired Dosage Volume (ml)	Desired Dosage Strength (IU)	Amount of Liquid to Add (ml)	Number of Doses That Will Result
10000	1.0	125	80.0	80.0
10000	1.0	133	75.2	75.2
10000	1.0	150	66.7	66.7
10000	1.0	166	60.2	60.2
10000	1.0	175	57.1	57.1
10000	1.0	200	50.0	50.0
10000	1.0	225	44.4	44.4
10000	1.0	250	40.0	40.0
10000	0.5	125	40.0	80.0
10000	0.5	133	37.6	75.2
10000	0.5	150	33.3	66.7
10000	0.5	166	30.1	60.2
10000	0.5	175	28.6	57.1
10000	0.5	200	25.0	50.0
10000	0.5	225	22.2	44.4
10000	0.5	250	20.0	40.0
5000	1.0	125	40.0	40.0
5000	1.0	133	37.6	37.6
5000	1.0	150	33.3	33.3
5000	1.0	166	30.1	30.1
5000	1.0	175	28.6	28.6
5000	1.0	200	25.0	25.0
5000	1.0	225	22.2	22.2
5000	1.0	250	20.0	20.0
5000	0.5	125	20.0	40.0
5000	0.5	133	18.8	37.6
5000	0.5	150	16.7	33.3
5000	0.5	166	15.1	30.1
5000	0.5	175	14.3	28.6
5000	0.5	200	12.5	25.0
5000	0.5	225	11.1	22.2
5000	0.5	250	10.0	20.0

Ampoule Size (IU)	Desired Dosage Volume (ml)	Desired Dosage Strength (IU)	Amount of Liquid to Add (ml)	Number of Doses That Will Result
2000	1.0	125	16.0	16.0
2000	1.0	133	15.0	15.0
2000	1.0	150	13.3	13.3
2000	1.0	166	12.0	12.0
2000	1.0	175	11.4	11.4
2000	1.0	200	10.0	10.0
2000	1.0	225	8.9	8.9
2000	1.0	250	8.0	8.0
2000	0.5	125	8.0	16.0
2000	0.5	133	7.5	15.0
2000	0.5	150	6.7	13.3
2000	0.5	166	6.0	12.0
2000	0.5	175	5.7	11.4
2000	0.5	200	5.0	10.0
2000	0.5	225	4.4	8.9
2000	0.5	250	4.0	8.0
1500	1.0	125	12.0	12.0
1500	1.0	133	11.3	11.3
1500	1.0	150	10.0	10.0
1500	1.0	166	9.0	9.0
1500	1.0	175	8.6	8.6
1500	1.0	200	7.5	7.5
1500	1.0	225	6.7	6.7
1500	1.0	250	6.0	6.0
1500	0.5	125	6.0	12.0
1500	0.5	133	5.6	11.3
1500	0.5	150	5.0	10.0
1500	0.5	166	4.5	9.0
1500	0.5	175	4.3	8.6
1500	0.5	200	3.8	7.5
1500	0.5	225	3.3	6.7
1500	0.5	250	3.0	6.0

Phase 2 Troubleshooting questions:

1. Did you use any nutritive oils or lotions on your skin?
2. Did you get any nutritive fats on your skin while preparing meals for others?
3. Did you eat chicken that is not breast meat or ground meat with added fillers or fat?
4. Did you eat any kind of turkey, any kind of smoked meat/fish, wrong types of fish?
5. Did you eat any meals out that might have had some unknown/hidden fat or sugar?
6. Are you cooking with Pam? Stop. It stalled one of the folks in my support group.
7. Are you using powdered Stevia that has maltodextrin or lactose in it? Change to liquid Stevia.
8. Are you using Equal (aspartame), Splenda (sucralose), or powdered Stevia packets that have maltodextrin or dextrose in it? Change to liquid Stevia.
9. Are you getting at least 8 hours of sleep per night, preferably continuous?
10. Did you take any pills that could have additives in them as fillers, or have a sugar coating?
11. Are you weighing your raw protein CAREFULLY for each/every meal?
12. Are you measuring your water to ensure intake of two liters or 64 ounces daily?
13. Are you only eating foods on Dr. Simeons' list? Sometimes, it helps to write out exactly what you ate and drank, to identify the problem.
14. Is it close to your menses or ovulation?
15. Are you at a weight that you maintained for an extended time in the past?

More suggestions to break a stall:

1. Drink MORE teas.
2. Try eating apples and ½ grapefruit instead of strawberries and oranges, which some stall on.
3. Try to walk at least a little more.
4. Try fresh spinach as your vegetable.
5. Cut out cabbage, which stalls some of us.
6. Eat nothing but organic.
7. Check your spice labels for hidden sugar or oil.
8. Drop the IM injection dosage to 125 IU. If that doesn't work, try increasing it in increments, but no more than 200 IU, unless injecting subcutaneous, and then the limit is 250 IU. Sublingual dosage should not exceed 333 IU per day, divided into 2 doses approximately 12 hours apart.
9. Start drinking an ACV cocktail 1-2 times per day.
10. Cut back on tomato consumption if you are eating them every day.
11. Cut back on shrimp consumption if you are eating them every day.
12. Try omitting the allowed Wasa/grissini/melba toast each day.
13. Try eating meals earlier in the day.
14. Eat at least one meal each day with a large green salad.
15. If you are drinking a gallon or more of water, drink less water, but at least 64 oz daily.
16. The detox baths suggested previously can help to break a stall sometimes.

Hang in there. I promise that you will start reducing again. Again, I learned everything that I needed to know about stalls in nursery school. "You get what you get and you don't get upset." I once stalled for 14 full days at a former long-term weight, just as Dr S says, and it ENDED just like he said it would. Yours will, too.

Pounds and Inches Tracking Chart

Date	Weight (lbs.)	Pounds change	Chest (in.)	Waist (in.)	Tummy (in.)	Hips (in.)	ThighL (in.)	ThighR (in.)	ArmL (in.)	ArmR (in.)	Total inches

Phase 3

Sugars

Which fruits are the "sweet fruits" that Dr. Simeons warned us to be careful with in Phase 3?

Based on glycemic impact, sweet fruits are considered to be any and all juiced, dried or dehydrated fruits because they become concentrated when fiber or all the liquid is removed as well as raw, fresh pomegranates, passion fruits, black currants, sweet cherries, bananas, dates, figs, mangoes, jackfruits, breadfruits, crabapples, cherimoyas, persimmons, prunes, raisins, and grapes.

Sugar or Starch Content and Glycemic Load

So many people think that Phase 3 is Atkins and that all carbs are starches or sugar. This is totally untrue. I must respectfully disagree with the assertion that " Carbohydrates = Starches and/or Sugars". While it is true that all sugar and starch are carbohydrates, all carbohydrates are NOT sugar and/or starch. Some carbohydrates are mostly fiber.

Because it is insulin release that allows fat to be stored in the body, I believe that Dr. S wanted patients to avoid high glycemic index foods during P3, although the term was not used back then. Glycemic index rates foods according to how likely that they are to cause blood sugar spikes and the resulting insulin release. To be clear, the current standard (since 1997) for glycemic effect (blood glucose raising potential) takes into consideration not only the GI rating, but also the amount of the serving, in order to estimate the total glycemic load (glycemic index times the carbohydrate content per serving size) based on both the quality and quantity of the food. If a standard serving of a food is larger, then that would raise the glycemic load, so both the amount and the GI rating of a food figure into whether you would eat it in P3, or if you need to strictly limit the serving size when you do eat it.

Phase 3 isn't Atkins induction, although some do use it as a rough guide. If it was, it wouldn't allow fruit. Dr. S only says to avoid the sweeter ones. You don't have to avoid all carbs. You simply do not eat refined sugar or starch at all. That being said, many Atkins recipes are good for Phase 3. Many non-Atkins recipes are, too, if they omit refined sugar and starch.

For example, some vegetables or grains are fibrous (non-starchy, mostly cellulose) and some are starchy. If you stick with fruits, vegetables, and grains with Glycemic Load under 4, you will have no problems, as long as you stay with a 3.5 ounce portion (100 grams). The portion size can change the Glycemic Load. For instance, if you eat 100 grams of hubbard squash, the Glycemic Load is 2, but if you eat 236 grams, it is 5.

To find the sugar or starch content or glycemic load of any food, use:

http://www.Nutritiondata.com or http://www.foodfacts.com.

Charts for Choosing P3 Foods

You won't see many processed foods on these charts because the emphasis should be on fresh whole foods, both in P3 and afterwards. Normally, a whole food would not have much sugar and it is naturally-occurring in a whole food, not added refined sugar.

Interestingly enough, some folks can't eat much fruit in P3 because of the sugar, even naturally-occurring, while others can eat bananas, which are not only very sweet fruit, which Simeons warns us to be careful with, but also depending on ripeness, may have some starch. As the fruit ripens, the starch turns to sugar.

We all seem to be different. Not only that, but each round of hCG seems to be a bit different from the last. Do the right thing by keeping good records and learning what works for you in

P3. That said, the first few days of P3, people seem more likely to have the violent fluctuations in weight that Dr. S referred to, that frequently do not happen with the same food in the last week of P3.

Any food listed as a "Maybe" for P3 should be used with caution and in very limited quantities, not more than 100 grams, which is what the Glycemic Load was based upon. You are more likely to have success with them after the first week of P3.

The first chart section lists food by whether or not it is suitable for P3, within each food category, to make it easy to choose P3-friendly foods. The second chart section lists food alphabetically within each food category to make it easy to find a particular food. Categories are fruits, vegetables or grains, protein, nuts, seeds, and miscellaneous.

P3 Charts Listing P3-Friendly Foods First

Type Of Fresh Raw Fruit	Sugar Content as % of Weight	Glycemic Load	Okay for P3?
Olive, black, ripe	0.0	1	Yes
Olive, green	0.5	1	Yes
Tomato	2.6	1	Yes
Oheloberry	Unk	1	Yes
Avocado	0.7	2	Yes
Lime	1.7	2	Yes
Lemon	2.5	2	Yes
Cranberry	4.0	2	Yes
Starfruit	4.0	2	Yes
Raspberry	4.4	2	Yes
Strawberry	4.9	2	Yes
Casaba Melon	5.7	2	Yes
Gooseberry	5.9	2	Yes
Papaya	5.9	2	Yes
Prickly Pear	6.0	2	Yes
Watermelon	6.2	2	Yes
Pear, Asian	7.0	2	Yes
Grapefruit, white	7.3	2	Yes
Honeydew Melon	8.1	2	Yes
Apple	10.4	3	Yes
Blackberry	4.9	3	Yes
Grapefruit, pink and red	6.9	3	Yes
Cantaloupe	7.9	3	Yes
Loganberry	8.0	3	Yes
Peach	8.4	3	Yes
Orange	9.4	3	Yes
Pear	9.8	3	Yes
Pineapple	9.8	3	Yes
Plum	9.9	3	Yes
Loquat	11.0	3	Yes
Blueberry	10.0	4	Maybe
Pineapple, extra sweet	10.3	4	Maybe
Mandarin Orange	10.6	4	Maybe
Tangerine	10.6	4	Maybe
Red Currant	7.4	4	Maybe
Mulberry	8.1	4	Maybe
Orange, navel	8.5	4	Maybe
Sour Cherry	8.5	4	Maybe
Guava (also starch)	8.9	4	Maybe
Kiwi (bit of starch)	9.0	4	Maybe

Type Of Fresh Raw Fruit	Sugar Content as % of Weight	Glycemic Load	Okay for P3?
Apricot	9.2	4	Maybe
Clementine	9.2	4	Maybe
Kumquat	9.4	4	Maybe
Elderberry	Unk	4	Maybe
Orange, Valencia	Unk	4	Maybe
Persimmon, Japanese	12.5	5	No
Sweet Cherry	12.8	5	No
Mango (also starch)	14.8	5	No
Passion Fruit	11.2	6	No
Pomegranate	13.7	6	No
Grape, seedless	15.5	6	No
Grape, sweet	16.2	6	No
Fig	16.3	6	No
Black Currant	Unk	6	No
Cherimoya	Unk	6	No
Crabapple	20.0	7	No
Banana (also starch)	12.2	8	No
Breadfruit	22.0	9	No
Jackfruits	22.0	10	No
Juice of any fruit	Varies	Varies	No
Persimmon, native	Unk	15	NO
Date, deglet noor	63.4	39	NO
Date, medjool	66.5	39	NO
Raisin	75.0	46	NO
Prune	89.0	57	NO

Type Of Vegetable or Grain	Starch Content as % of Weight	Glycemic Load	Okay for P3?
Endive	0	0	Yes
Sprouts, Alfalfa	0	0	Yes
Mustard Greens	2.1	0	Yes
Sour Pickles	2.3	0	Yes
Sprouts, mung bean	1.0	1	Yes
Olive, black, ripe	1.0	1	Yes
Watercress	1.3	1	Yes
Cucumber	2.2	1	Yes
Dill Pickle	2.6	1	Yes
Tomato	2.6	1	Yes
Olive, green	3.0	1	Yes

Type Of Vegetable or Grain	Starch Content as % of Weight	Glycemic Load	Okay for P3?
Rhubarb	3.0	1	Yes
Nopales	3.3	1	Yes
Lettuce	3.3	1	Yes
Summer Scallop Squash	3.4	1	Yes
Radish	3.5	1	Yes
Spinach	3.7	1	Yes
Summer Zucchini Squash	3.9	1	Yes
Celery	4.0	1	Yes
Green Pepper	4.2	1	Yes
Sauerkraut	4.3	1	Yes
Summer Crookneck or Straightneck Squash	4.3	1	Yes
Turnip Greens	4.4	1	Yes
Vegetable Juice, Canned	4.5	1	Yes
Jalapeno	4.7	1	Yes
Turnip	5.1	1	Yes
Avocado	0.7	2	Yes
Bamboo shoots	2.0	2	Yes
Arugula	3.7	2	Yes
Swiss Chard	4.1	2	Yes
Asparagus	4.1	2	Yes
Cauliflower	4.2	2	Yes
Radicchio	4.5	2	Yes
Collard Greens	4.9	2	Yes
Okra	4.9	2	Yes
Cabbage	5.5	2	Yes
Yellow Pepper	6.3	2	Yes
Winter Spaghetti Squash	6.5	2	Yes
Winter Hubbard Squash	6.5	2	Yes
Red Pepper	6.6	2	Yes
Leek	7.0	2	Yes
Yellow Onion	7.9	2	Yes
Pumpkin	8.1	2	Yes
Eggplant	8.1	2	Yes
Carrot	8.2	2	Yes
Beet greens	2.0	3	Yes
Dandelion greens	3.0	3	Yes
Parsley	3.0	3	Yes

Type Of Vegetable or Grain	Starch Content as % of Weight	Glycemic Load	Okay for P3?
Sprouts, kidney bean	4.0	3	Yes
String beans	4.0	3	Yes
Wax beans	4.0	3	Yes
Mushrooms (except Shiitake)	5.3	3	Yes
Kale	5.6	3	Yes
Kohlrabi	6.7	3	Yes
Snowpea	6.8	3	Yes
Brussels Sprout	7.1	3	Yes
Broccoli	7.2	3	Yes
Green Onion	7.3	3	Yes
Green Bean	7.9	3	Yes
Jicama	8.2	3	Yes
Globe Artichokes	12.0	3	Yes
Rutabagas	8.7	4	Maybe
White Onions	9.6	4	Maybe
Beets	10.0	4	Maybe
Winter Butternut Squash	10.5	4	Maybe
Water Chestnuts	12.3	4	Maybe
Winter Acorn Squash	14.6	4	Maybe
Sprouts, soybean	9.0	5	No
Shiitake Mushrooms	13.8	5	No
Broadbeans	10.1	6	No
Sprouts, pinto bean	12.0	6	No
Sprouts, navy bean	13.0	6	No
Hominy / Grits	14.3	6	No
English Peas	15.6	6	No
Parsnips	17.0	6	No
Lentils	19.5	6	No
Navy Beans	15.0	7	No
Jerusalem Artichokes	17.4	7	No
Sweet Potatoes	17.7	7	No
Bulgur Wheat	18.6	7	No
Split Peas	20.5	7	No
Lima Beans	20.9	7	No
Red Beans	21.8	7	No
Sweet Pickles	21.0	8	No

Type Of Vegetable or Grain	Starch Content as % of Weight	Glycemic Load	Okay for P3?
Black Beans	23.7	8	No
Potatoes	20.1	9	No
Quinoa	21.3	10	No
Sprouts, lentils	22.0	10	No
Brown Rice	23.0	11	No
Chickpeas (Garbanzo Beans)	27.4	10	No
Spelt	26.4	11	No
Yams	27.0	11	No
Couscous	23.2	12	NO
Corn	25.9	12	NO
Barley	28.2	12	NO
Pinto Beans	30.9	12	NO
Taro	34.6	14	NO
White Rice	28.2	15	NO
Spaghetti	30.6	16	NO
Whole Wheat English Muffins	40.4	18	NO
Whole Wheat Bread	41.3	19	NO
Yucca (Cassava)	38.1	20	NO
Sprouts, wheat	42.0	23	NO
Whole Wheat Rolls	51.1	26	NO
Whole Wheat Pita	55.0	27	NO
Whole Wheat Crackers	68.6	35	NO
Whole Buckwheat Groat Flour	70.6	37	NO
Oatmeal	69.0	39	NO
Millet	72.9	44	NO
Shredded Wheat, un-sweetened / sweetened	79.9/ 81.2	45/ 51	NO
Arrowroot Flour	88.1	59	NO

Type Of Protein/Fat	Sugar/Starch Content as % of Weight	Glycemic Load	Okay for P3?
Oil and Fats	0	0	Yes
Meat, poultry, seafood, or fish, grilled, fried in oil, baked, as long as it isn't breaded or cured meat such as ham, bacon if sugar-cured, hot dogs, or deli meat	0	0	Yes
Eggs (whole)	0	0	Yes
Cream, heavy whipping	3.0	0	Yes
Brie	0	0	Yes
Camembert	0	0	Yes
Gruyere	0	0	Yes
Cheddar	1.0	1	Yes
Colby	1.0	1	Yes
Cream Cheese, full-fat, no fillers	4.0	1	Yes
Roquefort	2.0	1	Yes
Cheddar	1.0	1	Yes
Edam	1.0	1	Yes
Muenster	1.0	1	Yes
Gouda	1.0	1	Yes
Cream, light whipping	3.0	1	Yes
Mozzarella	2.0	2	Yes
Blue cheese	2.0	2	Yes
Parmesan	2.0	2	Yes
Provolone	2.0	2	Yes
Romano	4.0	2	Yes
Swiss	5.0	2	Yes
Sour Cream	4.0	2	Yes
Half and Half	4.0	3	Yes
Yogurt (full fat)	5.0	3	Yes
Feta	4.0	3	Yes
Neufchatel	3.0	3	Yes
Ricotta, whole milk	3.0	3	Yes
Cottage cheese	3.0	3	Yes
Milk (whole)	5.0	4	Maybe
Buttermilk	5.0	4	Maybe
Tofu	Varies	Varies	No
Edamame	5.0	4	No
Low-fat Dairy	8.0	5	No

Type Of Protein/Fat	Sugar/Starch Content as % of Weight	Glycemic Load	Okay for P3?
Reduced-Fat Dairy	8.0	5	No
Non-fat Dairy	8.0	5	No
Velveeta cheese	10.0	5	No
American cheese	12.0	6	No

Type Of Raw Nuts	Sugar/Starch Content as % of Weight	Glycemic Load	Okay for P3?
Pine nuts	0.1	0	Yes
Tahini paste	0.5	0	Yes
Brazil nuts	0.7	0	Yes
Walnuts	0.7	0	Yes
Macadamia nuts	0.8	0	Yes
Coconut	0	2	Yes
Coconut milk	0	2	Yes
Pecans	1.5	0	Maybe
Hazelnuts	2.0	0	Maybe
Peanuts	6.0	0	Maybe
Almonds	2.7	1	Maybe
Peanut butter, natural, no sugar added	6.4	2	Maybe
Pistachio nuts	18.0	4	Maybe
Cashews	13.2	11	No
Chestnuts	29.6	21	No

Type of Seeds	Sugar/Starch Content as % of Weight	Glycemic Load	Okay for P3?
Flax seeds	0	0	Yes
Sesame seeds, dried and decorticated	0.5	0	Yes
Chia seeds	6.0	2	Yes
Sunflower seeds	16.3	0	Maybe
Watermelon seed kernels	15.3	2	Maybe
Pumpkin seed kernels (pepitas)	21.0	2	Maybe
Sesame seeds, if not dried and decorticated	10.0	8	No
Safflower seeds	34.0	16	No
Pumpkin seeds whole	54.0	34	No

Type Of Misc Food	Sugar/Starch Content as % of Weight	Glycemic Load	Okay for P3?
Capers	2.0	2	Yes
Horseradish	8.0	3	Yes
Mayonnaise, if homemade	0	0	Yes
Mustard	2.0	2	Yes
Vinegar, apple cider, red wine	1.0	0	Yes
Gravy, unless you make your own with konjac fiber	Varies	Varies	No
Vinegar, balsamic	17.0	6	No
Mayonnaise, if commercial, other than Duke's sugar free	24.0	9	No
Pudding of any kind	19.0	12	NO

P3 Quick Lookup Alphabetical Food Charts

Type Of Fresh Raw Fruit	Sugar Content as % of Weight	Glycemic Load	Okay for P3?
Apple	10.4	3	Yes
Apricot	9.2	4	Maybe
Avocado	0.7	2	Yes
Banana (also starch)	12.2	8	No
Black Currant	Unk	6	No
Blackberry	4.9	3	Yes
Blueberry	10.0	4	Maybe
Breadfruit	22.0	9	No
Cantaloupe	7.9	3	Yes
Casaba Melon	5.7	2	Yes
Cherimoya	Unk	6	No
Clementine	9.2	4	Maybe
Crabapple	20.0	7	No
Cranberry	4.0	2	Yes
Date, deglet noor	63.4	39	NO
Date, medjool	66.5	39	NO
Elderberry	Unk	4	Maybe
Fig	16.3	6	No
Gooseberry	5.9	2	Yes
Grape, seedless	15.5	6	No
Grape, sweet	16.2	6	No
Grapefruit, pink and red	6.9	3	Yes
Grapefruit, white	7.3	2	Yes
Guava (also starch)	8.9	4	Maybe
Honeydew Melon	8.1	2	Yes
Jackfruits	22.0	10	No
Juice of any fruit	Varies	Varies	No
Kiwi (bit of starch)	9.0	4	Maybe
Kumquat	9.4	4	Maybe
Lemon	2.5	2	Yes
Lime	1.7	2	Yes
Loganberry	8.0	3	Yes
Loquat	11.0	3	Yes
Mandarin Orange	10.6	4	Maybe
Mango (also starch)	14.8	5	No
Mulberry	8.1	4	Maybe
Oheloberry	Unk	1	Yes
Olive, black, ripe	0.0	1	Yes
Olive, green	0.5	1	Yes
Orange	9.4	3	Yes

Type Of Fresh Raw Fruit	Sugar Content as % of Weight	Glycemic Load	Okay for P3?
Orange, navel	8.5	4	Maybe
Orange, Valencia	Unk	4	Maybe
Papaya	5.9	2	Yes
Passion Fruit	11.2	6	No
Peach	8.4	3	Yes
Pear	9.8	3	Yes
Pear, Asian	7.0	2	Yes
Persimmon, Japanese	12.5	5	No
Persimmon, native	Unk	15	NO
Pineapple	9.8	3	Yes
Pineapple, extra sweet	10.3	4	Maybe
Plum	9.9	3	Yes
Pomegranate	13.7	6	No
Prickly Pear	6.0	2	Yes
Prune	89.0	57	NO
Raisin	75.0	46	NO
Raspberry	4.4	2	Yes
Red Currant	7.4	4	Maybe
Sour Cherry	8.5	4	Maybe
Starfruit	4.0	2	Yes
Strawberry	4.9	2	Yes
Sweet Cherry	12.8	5	No
Tangerine	10.6	4	Maybe
Tomato	2.6	1	Yes
Watermelon	6.2	2	Yes

Type Of Vegetable or Grain	Starch Content as % of Weight	Glycemic Load	Okay for P3?
Arrowroot Flour	88.1	59	NO
Arugula	3.7	2	Yes
Asparagus	4.1	2	Yes
Avocado	0.7	2	Yes
Bamboo shoots	2.0	2	Yes
Barley	28.2	12	NO
Beet greens	2.0	3	Yes
Beets	10.0	4	Maybe
Black Beans	23.7	8	No
Broadbeans	10.1	6	No
Broccoli	7.2	3	Yes
Brown Rice	23.0	11	No
Brussels Sprout	7.1	3	Yes

Type Of Vegetable or Grain	Starch Content as % of Weight	Glycemic Load	Okay for P3?
Bulgur Wheat	18.6	7	No
Cabbage	5.5	2	Yes
Carrot	8.2	2	Yes
Cauliflower	4.2	2	Yes
Celery	4.0	1	Yes
Chickpeas (Garbanzo Beans)	27.4	10	No
Collard Greens	4.9	2	Yes
Corn	25.9	12	NO
Couscous	23.2	12	NO
Cucumber	2.2	1	Yes
Dandelion greens	3.0	3	Yes
Dill Pickle	2.6	1	Yes
Eggplant	8.1	2	Yes
Endive	0	0	Yes
English Peas	15.6	6	No
Globe Artichokes	12.0	3	Yes
Green Bean	7.9	3	Yes
Green Onion	7.3	3	Yes
Green Pepper	4.2	1	Yes
Hominy / Grits	14.3	6	No
Jalapeno	4.7	1	Yes
Jerusalem Artichokes	17.4	7	No
Jicama	8.2	3	Yes
Kale	5.6	3	Yes
Kohlrabi	6.7	3	Yes
Leek	7.0	2	Yes
Lentils	19.5	6	No
Lettuce	3.3	1	Yes
Lima Beans	20.9	7	No
Millet	72.9	44	NO
Mushrooms (except Shiitake)	5.3	3	Yes
Mustard Greens	2.1	0	Yes
Navy Beans	15.0	7	No
Nopales	3.3	1	Yes
Oatmeal	69.0	39	NO
Okra	4.9	2	Yes
Olive, black, ripe	1.0	1	Yes
Olive, green	3.0	1	Yes
Parsley	3.0	3	Yes

127

Type Of Vegetable or Grain	Starch Content as % of Weight	Glycemic Load	Okay for P3?
Parsnips	17.0	6	No
Pinto Beans	30.9	12	NO
Potatoes	20.1	9	No
Pumpkin	8.1	2	Yes
Quinoa	21.3	10	No
Radicchio	4.5	2	Yes
Radish	3.5	1	Yes
Red Beans	21.8	7	No
Red Pepper	6.6	2	Yes
Rhubarb	3.0	1	Yes
Rutabagas	8.7	4	Maybe
Sauerkraut	4.3	1	Yes
Shiitake Mushrooms	13.8	5	No
Shredded Wheat, un-sweetened / sweetened	79.9/ 81.2	45/ 51	NO
Snowpea	6.8	3	Yes
Sour Pickles	2.3	0	Yes
Spaghetti	30.6	16	NO
Spelt	26.4	11	No
Spinach	3.7	1	Yes
Split Peas	20.5	7	No
Sprouts, Alfalfa	0	0	Yes
Sprouts, kidney bean	4.0	3	Yes
Sprouts, lentils	22.0	10	No
Sprouts, mung bean	1.0	1	Yes
Sprouts, navy bean	13.0	6	No
Sprouts, pinto bean	12.0	6	No
Sprouts, soybean	9.0	5	No
Sprouts, wheat	42.0	23	NO
String beans	4.0	3	Yes
Summer Crookneck or Straightneck Squash	4.3	1	Yes
Summer Scallop Squash	3.4	1	Yes

Type Of Vegetable or Grain	Starch Content as % of Weight	Glycemic Load	Okay for P3?
Summer Zucchini Squash	3.9	1	Yes
Sweet Pickles	21.0	8	No
Sweet Potatoes	17.7	7	No
Swiss Chard	4.1	2	Yes
Taro	34.6	14	NO
Tomato	2.6	1	Yes
Turnip	5.1	1	Yes
Turnip Greens	4.4	1	Yes
Vegetable Juice, Canned	4.5	1	Yes
Water Chestnuts	12.3	4	Maybe
Watercress	1.3	1	Yes
Wax beans	4.0	3	Yes
White Onions	9.6	4	Maybe
White Rice	28.2	15	NO
Whole Buckwheat Groat Flour	70.6	37	NO
Whole Wheat Bread	41.3	19	NO
Whole Wheat Crackers	68.6	35	NO
Whole Wheat English Muffins	40.4	18	NO
Whole Wheat Pita	55.0	27	NO
Whole Wheat Rolls	51.1	26	NO
Winter Acorn Squash	14.6	4	Maybe
Winter Butternut Squash	10.5	4	Maybe
Winter Hubbard Squash	6.5	2	Yes
Winter Spaghetti Squash	6.5	2	Yes
Yams	27.0	11	No
Yellow Onion	7.9	2	Yes
Yellow Pepper	6.3	2	Yes
Yucca (Cassava)	38.1	20	NO

Type Of Protein/Fat	Sugar/Starch Content as % of Weight	Glycemic Load	Okay for P3?
American cheese	12.0	6	No
Blue cheese	2.0	2	Yes
Brie	0	0	Yes
Buttermilk	5.0	4	Maybe
Camembert	0	0	Yes
Cheddar	1.0	1	Yes
Cheddar	1.0	1	Yes
Colby	1.0	1	Yes
Cottage cheese	3.0	3	Yes
Cream Cheese, full-fat, no fillers	4.0	1	Yes
Cream, heavy whipping	3.0	0	Yes
Cream, light whipping	3.0	1	Yes
Edam	1.0	1	Yes
Edamame	5.0	4	No
Eggs (whole)	0	0	Yes
Feta	4.0	3	Yes
Gouda	1.0	1	Yes
Gruyere	0	0	Yes
Half and Half	4.0	3	Yes
Low-fat Dairy	8.0	5	No
Meat, poultry, seafood, or fish, grilled, fried in oil, baked, as long as it isn't breaded or cured meat such as ham, bacon if sugar-cured, hot dogs, or deli meat	0	0	Yes
Milk (whole)	5.0	4	Maybe
Mozzarella	2.0	2	Yes
Muenster	1.0	1	Yes
Neufchatel	3.0	3	Yes
Non-fat Dairy	8.0	5	No
Oil and Fats	0	0	Yes
Parmesan	2.0	2	Yes
Provolone	2.0	2	Yes
Reduced-Fat Dairy	8.0	5	No
Ricotta, whole milk	3.0	3	Yes
Romano	4.0	2	Yes
Roquefort	2.0	1	Yes

Type Of Protein/Fat	Sugar/Starch Content as % of Weight	Glycemic Load	Okay for P3?
Sour Cream	4.0	2	Yes
Swiss	5.0	2	Yes
Tofu	Varies	Varies	No
Velveeta cheese	10.0	5	No
Yogurt (full fat)	5.0	3	Yes

Type Of Raw Nuts	Sugar/Starch Content as % of Weight	Glycemic Load	Okay for P3?
Almonds	2.7	1	Maybe
Brazil nuts	0.7	0	Yes
Cashews	13.2	11	No
Chestnuts	29.6	21	No
Coconut	0	2	Yes
Coconut milk	0	2	Yes
Hazelnuts	2.0	0	Maybe
Macadamia nuts	0.8	0	Yes
Peanut butter, natural, no sugar added	6.4	2	Maybe
Peanuts	6.0	0	Maybe
Pecans	1.5	0	Maybe
Pine nuts	0.1	0	Yes
Pistachio nuts	18.0	4	Maybe
Tahini paste	0.5	0	Yes
Walnuts	0.7	0	Yes

Type of Seeds	Sugar/Starch Content as % of Weight	Glycemic Load	Okay for P3?
Chia seeds	6.0	2	Yes
Flax seeds	0	0	Yes
Pumpkin seed kernels (pepitas)	21.0	2	Maybe
Pumpkin seeds whole	54.0	34	No
Safflower seeds	34.0	16	No
Sesame seeds, dried and decorticated	0.5	0	Yes
Sesame seeds, if not dried and decorticated	10.0	8	No
Sunflower seeds	16.3	0	Maybe
Watermelon seed kernels	15.3	2	Maybe

Type Of Misc Food	Sugar/Starch Content as % of Weight	Glycemic Load	Okay for P3?
Capers	2.0	2	Yes
Gravy, unless you make your own with konjac fiber	Varies	Varies	No
Horseradish	8.0	3	Yes
Mayonnaise, if commercial, other than Duke's sugar free	24.0	9	No
Mayonnaise, if homemade	0	0	Yes
Mustard	2.0	2	Yes
Pudding of any kind	19.0	12	NO
Vinegar, apple cider or red wine	1.0	0	Yes
Vinegar, balsamic	17.0	6	No

101 Names for Sugar

Typically, when ingredients are listed on a product, they must be listed from largest amount down to smallest amount found in that product. Do not be fooled into thinking there is very little sugar in an item if it is not listed near the beginning. Often you will find three or four of the following aliases in the ingredient listing, meaning that the product may be mostly sugar!

Added sugars in processed foods can be found under the following names:

1. Agave Syrup
2. Amasake
3. Any name ending in "ose" or "ol" or "syrup" (except for sucralose, which is Splenda)
4. Bar Sugar
5. Barbados Sugar
6. Barley Malt
7. Blackstrap Molasses
8. Black Sugar
9. Brown Sugar
10. Cane Juice
11. Cane Juice Crystals
12. Cane Sugar
13. Caramel
14. Caramel Coloring
15. Castor Sugar
16. Confectioner's Sugar
17. Corn Sweetener
18. Corn Syrup
19. Corn Syrup Solids
20. Crystallized Cane Juice
21. D-mannose
22. Date Sugar
23. Demerara
24. Demerara Sugar
25. Dehydrated Cane Juice

26. Dehydrated Cane Juice Crystals
27. Dextran
28. Dextrin
29. Dextrine
30. Dextrose (glucose)
31. Disaccharides
32. Evaporated Cane Juice
33. Evaporated Cane Juice Sugar
34. Florida crystals (a trademarked name)
35. Free Flowing Brown Sugars
36. Fructose
37. Fruit Juice Concentrate
38. Galactose
39. Galatactose
40. Glucose
41. Glucose Syrup
42. Golden Syrup
43. Granulated Sugar
44. Grape Sugar
45. Grape Sweetener
46. High Fructose Corn Syrup (HFCS)
47. Honey
48. Hydrolysed Starch
49. Hydrogenated Glucose Syrup
50. Hydrogenated Starch Hydrolysates (HSH)
51. Invert Sugar
52. Isomalt
53. Levulose
54. Lactitol
55. Lactose
56. Malt
57. Malt Extract
58. Malt Syrup
59. Maltodextrin
60. Maltitol
61. Maltose
62. Maple Syrup
63. Molasses

64. Monosaccharide
65. Muscovado
66. Organic Dehydrated Cane Juice
67. Panocha
68. Polysaccharide
69. Powdered Sugar
70. Rapadura
71. Raw Cane Crystals
72. Raw Honey
73. Raw Sugar
74. Refiner's Syrup
75. Ribose
76. Rice Extract
77. Rice Malt
78. Rice Syrup
79. Saccharide
80. Saccharose
81. Sorghum
82. Sorghum Syrup
83. Sucanat
84. Succanat
85. Sucrose
86. Sugar
87. Sweetener
88. Syrup
89. Table Sugar
90. Treacle
91. Turbinado
92. Turbinado Sugar
93. Unbleached Crystallized Evaporated Cane Juice
94. Unbleached Evaporated Sugar Cane Juice Crystals
95. Unbleached Sugar Cane
96. Unrefined Cane Juice Crystals
97. Washed Cane Juice Crystals
98. White Grape Juice
99. Yellow Sugar
100. Xylose
101. Xyulose

Phase 3 Sweeteners

The best alternatives to use for sweeteners in Phase 3 are:

- Stevia, a natural zero glycemic response sweetener
- Erythritol, a sugar alcohol with zero glycemic response
- Xylitol, another sugar alcohol with low glycemic response that can be used in small amounts to limit the digestive upset it can cause

I don't ever recommend artificial sweeteners such as:

- Sucralose: In a recent study by Duke University, rats that were fed Splenda (sucralose) for only three months gained 9%-12% more weight than those that were not. Even more frightening, those rats continued to gain more after the Splenda was discontinued. "Splenda Alters Gut Microflora and Increases Intestinal P-Glycoprotein and Cytochrome P-450 in Male Rats" Journal of Toxicology and Environmental Health Part A, vol. 71, No. 21, January 2008 http://tinyurl.com/DukeStudy

- Aspartame: Studies show it causes cancer in mice and rats http://tinyurl.com/aspartamestudy1 http://tinyurl.com/aspartamestudy2
- Saccharin: Dr Simeons allowed this one, but we now know it does indeed cause an insulin release just as sugar does http://tinyurl.com/SaccharinInsulin

Phase 3 Sample Menu

Here is a typical day in Phase 3 for me:

Breakfast

Coffee with cream

3 egg Omelet with 2 slices sharp cheese sometimes with homemade salsa or a veggie like asparagus or spinach

Pink Lady Apple with 1 Tablespoon Peanut Butter sometimes, but limit this, since it is 6.4% starch

Lunch

2 cups of homemade Chili with tomatoes and onions with cheese

Honeycrisp Apple or berries and whipping (heavy) cream

Coffee with cream

Dinner

Several (maybe 3) Tacos made with sour cream and salsa with cheese, wrapped in lettuce

Okra and Tomatoes (Rotel)

Homemade Cheesecake without sugar and no crust (one or two slices, depending on hunger)

Hot tea or cold sparkling water, sometimes flavored, sometimes with Stevia

Phase 4

After completing three weeks of no refined sugar or starches, you may proceed to Phase 4, very gradually adding small amounts of sugars and starches. Dr. Simeons requires three weeks of Phase 4 before beginning your second round of Phase 2, if needed. He assumed that people needing more than one round would do long rounds, rather than shorter 23-dose ones, but some have done serial short rounds to avoid immunity from the longer rounds. Dr Simeons stated on page 54: "Patients who need only 23 injections may be injected daily, including Sundays, as they never develop immunity."

Therefore, although P4 is increased on each subsequent round when doing rounds of 40 doses, for 23-dose rounds, 6 weeks (3 weeks of P3, 3 weeks of P4) is sufficient between each round.

Following is a handy table of how much time to use between the longer 40-dose rounds:

Between Rounds	Phase 3 (No sugar or starch)	Phase 4
1 and 2	3 weeks	3 weeks
2 and 3	3 weeks	5 weeks
3 and 4	3 weeks	9 weeks
4 and 5	3 weeks	17 weeks
5 and 6	3 weeks	23 weeks
Any subsequent rounds	3 weeks	23 weeks

The Rest of Your Life

Dr Simeons stated flat out that he only had a 70% long-term success rate. If you don't want to be part of the 30% that relapsed into obesity again, I believe that you must abandon most what you've been taught about nutrition and health for the past 30 years. Approach Phase 4, the rest of your life, as a great adventure in finding out just what you can eat and maintain, and in finding out how your appetite and food preferences have changed. Eating 40% fat, 30-40% protein, and 20-30% carbohydrates in my diet most days works for me. That is not to say that I don't eat more carbs on some days, but the day after, I return to those percentages. I thought about recommending that for everyone, but if there is one thing that I have learned in my support group, it is that we are all different. What I am reasonably sure about is what the optimum nutrition and healthy diet for you will NOT be:

- It will not be based upon avoiding cholesterol or eating low-fat or non-fat foods. None other than Dr Michael DeBakey said that in thousands, he had seen no significant, consistent correlation between cholesterol levels and arteriosclerosis.
  http://tinyurl.com/DeBakey
  http://tinyurl.com/DeBakey2
- It will not be based upon eating 6 to 11 servings of grains per day, and correspondingly less fat, which was a government experiment (the food pyramid) gone horribly wrong. Harvard School of Public Health reported that when we were eating 45% fat, 13% were obese and less than 1% had diabetes. Reducing the fat to 33% resulted in 34% obesity rates and 8% diabetes incidence. Do you think that's a coincidence? I don't.
  http://tinyurl.com/PerCentFat

Final Tribute to Dr. Simeons

I would like to conclude this book with a commemorative link to a photo of Dr Alfred Theodore William Simeons' gravestone at Acattolico Cemetery (the old cemetery for non-Catholic foreigners) in Rome:

http://tinyurl.com/SimeonsGrave

When you see what this diet does for you, Dr Simeons will mean something very special and precious to you as he does to me.

Also by Harmony Clearwater Grace

HCG Diet Made Simple

The HCG Diet Book of Secrets

www.ingramcontent.com/pod-product-compliance
Lightning Source LLC
Chambersburg PA
CBHW070807280326
41934CB00012B/3101